# What Every Home Health Nurse Needs to Know

## A Book of Readings

# What Every Home Health Nurse Needs to Know

## A Book of Readings

Edited by
Marjorie McHann, RN, BS
Memphis, Tennessee

CONSULTANTS IN CARE / Memphis, Tennessee

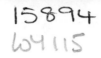

*Editor:*  Marjorie McHann, RN, BS
*Associate Editor:*  Dorothy Lambert, RN
*Copy Editor:*  Leigh Powell
*Design:*  Nikki Schroeder
*Production:*  John Bottenfield

Copyright © 1994
Consultants in Care
540 South Mendenhall Road #12-250
Memphis, Tennessee  38117

Notice:  The editor and publisher of this book have taken care that the information and recommendations contained herein are accurate and compatible with the standards generally accepted at the time of publication.

**Library of Congress Cataloging-in-Publication Data**

McHann, Marjorie.
   What every home health nurse needs to know: A book of readings.

Library of Congress Catalogue Card Number:  94-94127
ISBN Number:  0-9640767-0-5

PRINTED IN THE UNITED STATES OF AMERICA

To Mike

# Contributors

American Journal of Nursing Co.
555 West 57th Street
New York, New York  10019
(212)582-8820

American Nurses Association
600 Maryland Avenue SW #100 W
Washington, DC  20024
(202)544-4444

Aspen Publishers, Inc.
200 Orchard Ridge Drive #200
Gaithersburg, Maryland  20878
(301)417-7500

Health Standards & Quality Bureau
6325 Security Boulevard
Baltimore, Maryland  21207
(410)966-1366

J.B. Lippincott Company
227 East Washington Square
Philadelphia, Pennsylvania  19106
(215)238-4361

C.J. Humphrey & P. Milone-Nuzzo
c/o Appleton & Lange
25 Van Zant Street
East Norwalk, Connecticut  06855
(203)838-4400

Medical Economics Publishing
5 Paragon Drive
Montvale, NJ  07645
(201)358-4314

National Association for Home Care
519 C Street, NE, Stanton Park
Washington, DC  20002
(202)547-7424

Nursing Videos
540 South Mendenhall Road #12-250
Memphis, Tennessee  38117
(800)998-1945

S-N Publications, Inc.
103 North Second Street
Dundee, Illinois  60118
(708)426-6100

# Contents

*Preface* . . . . . . . . . . . . . . . . . . . . . . . . . . . . . . . . . . . . . . . . . . . .  xi

**CHAPTER 1.    MEDICARE COVERAGE ISSUES** . . . . . . . . . . . . .    1
Orientation to Home Care:  Maximizing Medicare Reimbursement    3
Management and Evaluation . . . . . . . . . . . . . . . . . . . . . . . . .   13
Medicare Guidelines Regarding Patient Teaching  . . . . . . . . . . . .   17
Home Care Strictly by the Rules . . . . . . . . . . . . . . . . . . . . . . .   27
The Denial Dilemma  . . . . . . . . . . . . . . . . . . . . . . . . . . . . . .   31

**CHAPTER 2.    SKILLED DOCUMENTATION** . . . . . . . . . . . . .   35
Charting that makes it through the Medicare Maze . . . . . . . . . .   37
Home Care Charting Dos and Don'ts . . . . . . . . . . . . . . . . . . .   41
Visit Notes . . . . . . . . . . . . . . . . . . . . . . . . . . . . . . . . . . . .   47
Documentation in Home Care:  Skilled Observation . . . . . . . . .   51
Documentation in Home Care:  Teaching . . . . . . . . . . . . . . . .   55
Skilled Nursing HCFA-485 and HCFA-486 Tips  . . . . . . . . . . . .   61

**CHAPTER 3.    CLINICAL MANAGEMENT** . . . . . . . . . . . . . . .   67
The Qualities of a Home Health Care Nurse . . . . . . . . . . . . . .   69
Home Visiting Steps . . . . . . . . . . . . . . . . . . . . . . . . . . . . . .   79
Priorities . . . . . . . . . . . . . . . . . . . . . . . . . . . . . . . . . . . . . .   87
Productivity  . . . . . . . . . . . . . . . . . . . . . . . . . . . . . . . . . . . .   91
Discharge Planning . . . . . . . . . . . . . . . . . . . . . . . . . . . . . . .   97
Two Halves Don't Make a Whole . . . . . . . . . . . . . . . . . . . . . .  101
Evaluation of the Therapeutic Nurse-Patient Relationship . . . . .  103
The Home Care Nurse as Case Manager . . . . . . . . . . . . . . . . .  107

**CHAPTER 4.    PATIENT EDUCATION** ................... **113**
Successful Client Teaching - What Makes the Difference? ..... 115
Helping Older Learners Learn .......................... 119
Patient Education: Motivating the Learner ................ 125
Health Teaching: The Crux of Home Care Nursing .......... 129
Needs to Know, Wants to Know, Ought to Know ............ 133

**CHAPTER 5.    QUALITY ASSURANCE ISSUES** ............ **135**
Quality Assurance in Home Care Services ................. 137
Patient Complaints ................................... 145
How to Promote Patient Satisfaction ..................... 149
Discharge Planning and Quality Assurance ................ 153

**CHAPTER 6.    LEGAL ISSUES** ........................ **157**
Legal Implications of Home Health Care .................. 159
Can You Meet the National Standard of Care in Home Health
Nursing? ........................................... 167
Documenting Patient Care in the Home - Legal Issues for Home
Health Nurses ...................................... 171
Avoiding Professional Negligence: A Review .............. 177
Delegation and Supervision of Patient Care ............... 183

**APPENDICES** ....................................... **187**
Appendix A.   Homecare Bill of Rights ................... 189
Appendix B.   Generic Quality Screens - Home Health Agency . 193
Appendix C.   The ANA Home Care Nursing Standards ...... 197

# Preface

Despite the rapid growth and changes occurring in the home health field, it's generally recognized that the existing literature for home health nurses falls far behind. This is especially evident to me as a consultant. Oftentimes I refer home health nurses to a myriad of hard to find journal articles, videos, and books that provide the kind of practical, down-to-earth information they need every day.

For this reason, I decided to edit this book, combining these often recommended readings into one source of pertinent, practical information for home health nurses. **What Every Home Health Nurse Needs to Know** was edited with "new" home health nurses in mind, but experienced practicing home health nurses will also benefit from the book, and nurses involved in administrative and educational aspects of agency operation will find it a useful resource for orientation and clinical support purposes.

This book is organized into six chapters:

- Chapter 1 reviews the skilled nursing services covered by Medicare.
- Chapter 2 discusses proper documentation of HCFA Forms 485/486 and skilled nursing visit notes to maximize reimbursement.
- Chapter 3 review concepts pertinent to nursing practice within the patient's home environment.
- Chapter 4 includes readings on several important aspects of the teaching/learning process.
- Chapter 5 discusses important issues of quality assurance specific to home health nursing practice.
- Chapter 6 contains meaningful insights on important legal issues specific to home health nursing.

**What Every Home Health Nurse Needs to Know** addresses both the science and the sensitivity integral to home health nursing. It's my hope that nurses will find it a useful resource as they face the special challenges of nursing practice in the home setting.

---

——————————————————————————CHAPTER 1

# Medicare Coverage
# Issues

# Orientation to Home Care: Maximizing Medicare Reimbursement

*Joan Evelyn Johnston, PhD, RN, GNP*
*Betty R. Clark, RN, MEd*

In an age of Medicare denials for payment of home health services, nurses must carefully examine their care to make sure that nursing and other services are necessary, effective, and reimbursable.[1-3] In this climate of uncertainty, nurses ask, "What can I do to be sure my home care will be appropriate and payable by Medicare?" This question should be asked during the intake process, because after care has been provided, a denial could come from the Medicare fiscal intermediary stating that skilled care was not necessary, and all visits made could be non-covered. Nurses should check the appropriateness of their care, not only at admission, but during the entire service period to ensure that documentation reflects payability.

## SOURCE OF REGULATIONS

A number of governmental agencies have written regulations that specify how home nursing care is to be given (Table 1). First, the legislation enacted as Medicare Title XVIII, Social Security Act (1966), is further defined by the Code of Federal Regulations (CFR) in the *Federal Register.* The CFR regulations are then further defined by the federal Health Care Financing Administration (HCFA) in the *Medicare Home Health Agency Manual.*[4] This document, which will be referred to as HIM-11, is the home care nurse's bible for reimbursement.

The HCFA has regional offices throughout the United States,

and supervises payments through the so-called fiscal intermediary (FI) which the HCFA selects for each region.[5] FIs are private insurance companies that actually do the payment review for Medicare, and either send the home care agency a check or deny payment.[6] Not only must nurses be concerned with the federal regulations in CFR and HIM-11, they also must review two other guidelines: transmittals from HCFA summarizing updates to HIM-11, and newsletters from the regional FI, which further interpret the federal regulations. These newsletters come to the home health agency on a continuing basis, and may differ from region to region. This pyramid of regulations may seem confusing, but essentially the nurse needs to look at only four documents: the CFR, HIM-11, transmittals from HCFA, and newsletters from the regional FI. Failure to stay updated on these documents is a sure way to fail to be reimbursed for services.

## ADMISSION TO SERVICES

There are four eligibility criteria that must be considered before a patient is admitted to a home health service.[7] The nurse, physical therapist, or speech pathologist must go through the following thought processes when the physician orders home care:

1. *Is the service skilled?* To determine if the service is skilled, the nurse, physical therapist, or speech pathologist assesses the condition of the patient and the complexity of the services.[8] The question must be asked: Could the average nonmedical person provide these services? For example, a nonmedical person would not know how to insert a catheter or teach gait training for walker ambulation. Remember, the service is not skilled just because it is performed by a licensed professional.[8] The skills of a nurse are not required to give an enema since the average nonmedical person already has the knowledge or expertise to render this service, and a prepackaged prepared solution can be purchased over the counter. When a patient has been cleaning and changing his own tracheostomy for two months, it is not necessary to have the nurse teach or perform this procedure unless further illness or complication has occurred. If a competent person is not available to perform a non-skilled service, it does not become skilled just because the nurse or therapist performs it.[8] If a patient only needs a clean dressing over a nondraining wound for protection, and she is unable to carry out this for herself, it is not skilled for the nurse to dress this wound.

**Table 1. Government Pyramid of Regulations for Home Health Agencies.**

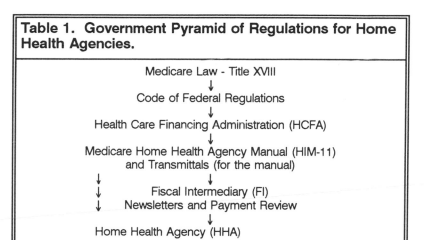

Medicare Law - Title XVIII
↓
Code of Federal Regulations
↓
Health Care Financing Administration (HCFA)
↓
Medicare Home Health Agency Manual (HIM-11)
and Transmittals (for the manual)
↓                    ↓
↓           Fiscal Intermediary (FI)
↓      Newsletters and Payment Review
↓
Home Health Agency (HHA)

2. *Is the patient homebound?* This does not mean the patient has to be bedbound. Answers to the following questions can be helpful in establishing the homebound status. Does the patient still drive to appointments? If so, the patient is not homebound. Where does the patient go? If the answer is to church, shops, or social events -- on a routine basis even though accompanied by another person or supportive device -- this patient would not be considered homebound. Is it a "considerable and taxing effort?"[9] In other words, does the absence from home put a physiological demand on the condition of the injury or illness, or even worsen the condition? Would the patient suffer from dyspnea, chest pain, or fluctuation of vital signs if he or she left home for nonmedical reasons? Even if the patient goes to the physician several times within a month, the homebound status could be questioned. Is the patient able to seek health services outside the home? The homebound status not only has to be certified by the physician in the plan of treatment and described in the monthly update for reimbursement, but also must be clearly documented throughout the progress notes, although not necessarily on each note. Again it may depend on your FI.

3. *Is the care intermittent?* Assess this point by asking: Is there a recurring, medically predictable need?[10] Can it be expected that the condition will change within a specified period? Is the care ordered daily? If so, remember to obtain documentation from the physician on how long the daily visits are expected to be needed.

Intermittent care usually means several times a week for 60 days or less.

4. *What is the medical need?* Is it medically necessary and reasonable? The plan of treatment and the nursing care plan must reflect the patient's need. Does the patient have a new diagnosis or an exacerbation of an existing diagnosis? Can you see a "desired result"?[9] Can the patient's needs be met in the home setting? Is the required care skilled or custodial?

When a referral is received, the nurse must contact the physician and discuss the specific orders for care. These orders must include types and frequency of services, medical diagnoses (not symptoms), functional limitations, current medications (noting if they are new or changed), prescribed diet, and medical supplies. While you have the physician's attention, attempt to get as much medical history and clinical findings as you can. This information will make your initial visit more comfortable for both the patient and you. Some physicians are not familiar with the Medicare rules and regulations, so usually it is up to the nurse to explain these.[11] One of the areas that usually is unclear to the physician is how to determine the frequency of visits. The physician has to agree to a specific frequency as the nurse assesses it on the initial visit, based on the condition of the patient and the needed interventions. Remember, frequency can be changed, and should be when the patient's condition changes.

## FREQUENCY OF VISITS

One way to determine the frequency of visits is to assess the nursing interventions needed to obtain a specific goal (a desired result). If the patient does not require hands-on treatment and only needs observation and evaluation, then frequent visits are ordered for short duration. For example, the patient has a long history of hypertension and recently had an exacerbation -- elevated blood pressure. The physician prescribed a new antihypertensive and diuretic and ordered home care. The frequency of visits could generally be for several times a week for 3 or 4 weeks. This allows time for the nurse to assess the effectiveness of the new medications and observe vital signs and other symptoms of hypertension for stability. If the patient had side effects from the new medications, or they were not effective, then the nurse would report this. The physician would probably make another change in the medication regime and the frequency would be extended for another 3 weeks for observation and evaluation.

In determining the number of teaching visits, consideration must be given to whether the teaching provided constitutes follow-up of teaching given in the hospital or is the initial instruction received by the patient. For example, a new insulin-dependent diabetic will receive limited instruction in the hospital, and will need additional teaching in the home setting. Daily visits to teach and assess the injection technique and diabetic care would be reasonable for 7 to 10 days and might even extend slightly beyond that time frame. Visits made solely to emphasize or to remind the patient to follow instructions do not require the skills of a nurse. It is much easier to determine a frequency when the physician orders specific treatments, like wound care or catheter changes. Again, you might have to educate the physician on what Medicare will reimburse for these treatments. A reasonable frequency for wound care could be daily for several weeks depending upon the stage and seriousness of the wound (with the proper medical documentation). During these visits, you should be teaching wound care to the patient or caregiver or both. Your documentation should reflect the character, location, drainage, size of the wound, dressing materials, and technique used, and should also note the healing process and the response to treatment.

## REFERRALS TO OTHER DISCIPLINES

Referrals to services other than nursing occur as a result of the assessment process. Could the patient benefit from restorative interventions of a physical therapist (PT), occupational therapist (OT), or speech pathologist (SP)? Is it expected that the patient will improve significantly in a reasonable period of time? During the initial visit, the PT, OT, or SP will make an assessment of the medical need, rehabilitation potential, and specific modalities needed to obtain the optimum level of function. Then a course of intervention will be planned and implemented.

There are other services that need to be considered besides those skilled services of the nurse, PT, OT, and SP. Home health aide services can be ordered by the physician if patients are unable to provide their own personal care. The services of a home health aide can be provided only while patients are receiving skilled services. Another service within this same guideline is that of medical social worker. A social worker referral is made only when social problems are interfering with the "patient's medical condition or his rate of recovery".[12] The duration allowed for social services is often minimal, and justified to diagnose emotional or social conditions that may be inhibiting the treatment plan.

## EQUIPMENT NEEDS

Another area to consider at the initial visit or at subsequent visits is the need for durable medical equipment. Whether the home health agency supplies it or refers to a local equipment company, the patient should be involved in the equipment order. If patients have qualifying diagnoses for specific types of equipment, they should be informed of the cost and their obligations for payment. Equipment can be rented or purchased, and this usually depends on whether the equipment will be used temporarily or permanently.[13] Do not assume that Medicare will pay for equipment just because the physician has ordered it. If you have questions regarding reimbursement for equipment, contact the FI or an equipment company.[2]

## DOCUMENTATION

Information on admission criteria and the plan of treatment is documented on printed governmental forms. Each agency has its own nurses' or therapy progress forms on which a visit is documented. Whether the note is documented on a checklist or as a narrative note, it must reflect the plan of treatment as ordered. Every note should be able to stand alone. It should contain the homebound status, the clinical picture based on subjective and objective observations, and the skilled intervention that was rendered. It must match the plan of treatment. Questions to ask are: Was there reason to contact the physician? Is service covered (reimbursable) care? Medicare will not pay for services if they are directed toward prevention, and certain words or phrases can also cause a denial of payment. For example, the patient's condition is *stable,* the patient was *not at home,* or previous teaching was *reviewed, reinforced or repeated.*[14] Also, it is not considered a reimbursable intervention to provide only emotional support to a terminally ill patient.

Once a note is completed, it should be carefully reviewed. Does it contain the response to teaching? Does it show continuity of care? Is there a reason to increase or decrease the frequency of visits? Are there new patient problems? It may be time-consuming to answer all of these questions on each note, but one note can get the entire length of stay denied.[15]

## DISCHARGE FROM SERVICE

The length of time a patient stays on service is determined by many individual factors as well as general practice, which indicates how long certain types of patients may receive care. Visits can be made to patients as long as those visits are "reasonable and necessary to the *treatment*" of the patient's illness or injury and are based on "*medical need.*"[16]

To assess the need for discharge ask the following questions:

1. Can the visits be documented as skilled by the guidelines?
2. Can the frequency and duration of visits be justified?
3. Do the nurse's notes reflect that the patient is making steady progress toward the goals in the plan of care? (Maintenance of chronic conditions is *not* reimbursable.)
4. If steady progress is not evident, has a new condition occurred that would qualify the patient for more skilled visits?
5. Has the physician changed the plan of treatment so further skilled nursing observation is needed?
6. Does the patient still meet the qualifications for admission to service? Any change in these (eg, homebound status) could mean payment will be denied.

Certain patients can be seen for a long period of time if they meet the "requirement for intermittent skilled nursing care," which is defined as "medically predictable recurring needs."[10] Ordinarily such a patient would need to be seen at least once every 30 days. These patients typically are those with urinary catheters, feeding tubes, and/or repeated blood work (eg, warfarin levels).

Patients seen less often than every 30 days must have justification of recurring medical need for skilled nursing service. Again, monitoring of chronic conditions is not justified, *unless a medically predictable* need can be foreseen. Examples given by HIM-11[10] are patients who (1) have a silicone catheter that is changed every 90 days, (2) have fecal impactions that require manual removal, and (3) are blind diabetics who self-inject insulin and need observation to determine if a change in the type or level of care is needed (as a *supplement* to physician's contacts with the patient, not as a replacement for them).

Discharge planning begins at admission by determining the reasonable and practical goals the patient should achieve. During all visits, the nurse incorporates plans for discharge by initiating referrals for support systems that the patient and family will use to continue maintenance of health after home visits end.

Plans for discharge from service are discussed with patients and their families during the admission visit so that they will have a realistic expectation of what the nursing agency can provide. Plans for care are directed toward a gradual increase in the patients' and caregivers' ability to take over patient care, and thus no longer need home visits. Team conferences of all disciplines involved should be documented, illustrating coordination of care and the progress of patients toward the goals set; thus, progress toward discharge.[17]

An understanding of the nurse-patient relationship also begins at admission. The patient and family need a reasonable time-frame and an assurance that needed nursing care will be provided, but they must be encouraged not to become dependent on the nurse. Provisions of Medicare reimbursement need to be carefully explained to the patient and family so they will understand when and under what circumstances home care will end.[7]

As the discharge date approaches, the patient and family need to be reassessed for further needs not present at admission. More skilled visits can be offered if untoward clinical findings occur; however, these must be justified under the HIM-11 guidelines.[16] If additional referrals are needed, these should be made the same day they are recognized to assure that services are obtained and satisfactory to the patient and family before discharge. Finally, patients and families need to be encouraged to call the home health agency for follow-up care or possible readmission to service if changes in need occur.

## A FINAL WORD

Nurses' natural inclinations are to provide good nursing care to anyone who needs it regardless of ability to pay. It is really not necessary to deny needed care to patients;[18] it *is* necessary to search the Medicare manual (HIM-11) to find the guideline that best suits the patients' need for *skilled* services. Agencies usually develop the internal clinical experience to accomplish this and can always consult with the nurse from their FI. If you have a belief that the patient needs skilled care, it is probably true. Analyze the data for needs that are recognized in the guidelines. While providing reimbursable skilled care, remember, there is no reason why you cannot provide for other needs as well. Keep in mind that Medicare is an insurance program that covers an intensive level of home care. Comprehensive nursing care can and should be given. Knowing the Medicare guidelines thoroughly most often leads to justification for skilled care.

---

## REFERENCES

1. Connaway N: Documenting patient care in the home: Legal issues for home health nurses. *Home Healthcare Nurse* 1985; 3(5): 6-8.
2. Curtiss FR: Recent developments in federal reimbursement for home health care. *Am J Hosp Pharm* 1986; 43(1): 132-9.
3. Reif L: Making dollars and sense of home health policy. *Nurse Economics* 1984; 2(6): 382-388.
4. Health Care Financing Administration: *Medicare Home Health Agency Manual*. HCFA publication No. HIM-11, Sec 200. Washington, DC: Superintendent of Documents, 1986.
5. O'Malley ST: Reimbursement issues. In: Stuart-Siddall S (ed): *Home Health Care Nursing*, Rockville, Md: Aspen Systems, 1986, pp. 23-82.
6. Health Care Financing Administration: *Medicare Program*: Assignment and reassignment of home health agencies to designated regional intermediaries. *Federal Register* 1985; 50: 14162-5.
7. Humphrey CJ: *Home Care Nursing Handbook*, Norwalk, Conn: Appleton-Century-Crofts, 1986.
8. Health Care Financing Administration: *Medicare Home Health Agency Manual*. HCFA publication No. HIM-11, Sec 204.2 AM-D. Washington, DC: Superintendent of Documents, 1986.
9. Health Care Financing Administration: *Medicare Home Health Agency Manual*. HCFA publication No. HIM-11, Sec 208.4. Washington, DC: Superintendent of Documents, 1986.
10. Health Care Financing Administration: *Medicare Home Health Agency Manual*. HCFA Pub. No. HIM-11, Sec. 204.1. Washington, DC: Superintendent of Documents, 1986.
11. Hansen JW: Future trends in home health care. In: Stuart-Siddall S (ed): *Home Health Care Nursing*, Rockville, Md: Aspen Systems, 1986, pp. 23-82.
12. Health Care Financing Administration: *Medical Home Health Agency Manual*. HCFA publication No. HIM-11, Sec 106.1. Washington, DC: Superintendent of Documents, 1986.
13. Health Care Financing Administration: *Durable Medical Equipment:* Making the Rental/Purchase Decision. HFCA publication No. HIM-14.3, Sec 41060. Washington, DC: Superintendent of Documents, 1986.
14. Holloway, VM: Documentation: One of the ultimate challenges in home health care, *Home Healthcare Nurse*, 1984; 2(1): 19,22.
15. Hoffman J: Compliance audit. *Home Health J* (September) 1984:21.
16. Health Care Financing Administration: *Medicare Home Health Agency Manual*. HCFA publication No. HIM-11, Sec 203.3. Washington, DC: Superintendent of Documents, 1986.
17. Stanhope M, Sheahan S, Kent E: The community health nurse as client advocate. In: Stanhope M. Lancaster J (eds): *Community Health Nursing: Process and Practice for Promoting Health*, ed 2. St Louis: CV Mosby, 1988, pp. 744-61.
18. Alper PR: Medicare games just get sillier and sillier. *Med Economics* (March) 1985: 131-135.

# Management and Evaluation

*Pat Carr, RN*

Copyright 1990 J.B. Lippincott Company.
Reprinted from *Home Healthcare Nurse,* Vol 8, Num 5.
Used with permission. All rights reserved.

Home health nurses have always acted as managers of patient care. We have always worked with other disciplines and caregivers to assess the care delivered and make changes as necessary. This function has always been part of the job, although it was never recognized as a skilled nursing activity by HCFA.

Recent revisions to the HIM-11 have recognized the skill involved in managing and evaluating a patient care plan, and it is now a reimbursable nursing function. Now the ball is back in our court. Now we have to define management and evaluation, select appropriate patients, and develop adequate documentation.

Defining the skill should be simple. After all, we do it every day on a majority of patients. Yet there is a problem. Nurses who do home health are geared to looking at reimbursable nursing services as active services. We do procedures. We teach caregivers. Historically, we are more comfortable with the hands-on care we deliver. Our documentation is directed toward active skills. Now we have to define as a reimbursable skill an activity that is a gray area. We have to define the process of assessing the spectrum of care a patient is receiving, evaluating the effectiveness of that care, and making the necessary changes.

The HIM-11 revision of July 1989 defines management and evaluation of a patient care plan in the following manner;

*"For skilled nursing care to be reasonable and necessary for management and evaluation of the beneficiary's plan of care, the complexity of the necessary unskilled services which are a necessary*

*part of the medical treatment must require the involvement of skilled
nursing personnel to promote the patient's recovery and medical safety
in view of the beneficiary's overall condition."*

For those of us looking at actual patients, the above definition
is a little wordy to carry around. We can define management and
evaluation as simply the process of monitoring and altering the
unskilled patient services to ensure the patient's safety, progress,
and ability to stay at home. The unskilled services may include
those provided by a home health aide, family member, or
companion. Nutrition, skin care, exercise, and assistance with
bowel function may be some of the services provided. We can also
define the skill by setting criteria for the selection of patients.

The patient requiring management and evaluation has very
limited mobility and is dependent on caregivers for much of his
personal care. He has a diagnosis or multiple diagnoses that put
him at risk for complications. An example would be the patient
with COPD, osteoporosis, and fragile skin secondary to steroid
therapy. The patient with severe Parkinsonism, difficulty in eating,
and chronic constipation due to medication might also need
management and evaluation.

We can also set criteria for patient selection by using our
experience with patients. Look closely at the patients who require
a great deal of unskilled care and whose activity is very limited. In
this group, who are the patients whom we hate to discharge
because we know they will be back on service in six weeks with a
recurrence of the original problem? Who are the patients with
Foley catheters who are constantly requiring extra visits because
their catheters are plugged due to poor hydration? Who are the
patients who we know are going to experience skin breakdown
because they are skill bedbound six weeks after a CVA? Who are
the patients who require unskilled care that needs to be
periodically evaluated by a professional to maintain medical safety?
It may be difficult at first to identify the patients at risk and to set
criteria. We can best proceed by using our experience, our
common sense, and our understanding that certain patients have
unskilled care needs that affect their medical status.

Once we have identified the patients who qualify for
management and evaluation services, how do we document the
care? Again, we are traditionally accustomed to dealing with acute
situations, and our documentation is more heavily geared to action
than to assessment. Yet every time we enter a home to see a
patient, we bring to that home a knowledge base and an

understanding of the importance of unskilled services to that patient's progress. Now we have to write it down. We have to be aware that for the patient under management and evaluation, our notes should reflect a precise assessment of the care that the patient is currently receiving, as well as the standard assessment of the patient's condition. We must document our evaluation of the care and any changes that we make in that care. We must remember that our visits are made to evaluate care, not caregivers. Documentation should also include communication with other disciplines providing services, as well as other caregivers.

The skill of management and evaluation of a patient care plan is not new. The only thing that is new is the recognition by HCFA that management and evaluation is a reimbursable skill. It may very well become the most valuable service that home health agencies can provide. Historically, home health nurses have entered acute situations, put out fires, and walked out the door. Now, we have an opportunity to continue service after the acute flames are out, and possibly do some fire prevention. That is progress. All we have to do is learn to use it.

# Medicare Guidelines Regarding Patient Teaching

*J.E. Jackson*
*E.A. Johnson*

Reprinted from *Patient Education in Home Care*
by J.E. Jackson and E.A. Johnson, pp. 51-60,
with permission of Aspen Publishers, Inc., © 1988.

## INTRODUCTION

Home health care became eligible for Medicare reimbursement with the creation of Medicare in 1965. The Medicare program provides reimbursement for care rendered by licensed nurses, physical therapists, speech pathologists, occupational therapists, medical social workers, and home health aides only under very specific and often times very limited circumstances. Not every Medicare beneficiary meets the criteria necessary to qualify for home health services coverage. Although it is recognized that services of an unskilled nature may be beneficial and of great importance to patients in their attempts to maintain, as much as possible, a normal existence at home, unskilled types of services are not covered under existing Medicare program regulations except as an extension of a skilled service, e.g., occupational therapy and home health aides.

It should be emphasized that Medicare does not provide coverage for general health care guidance, maintenance services, preventative illness training, and in general, the meeting of socioeconomic or emotional needs of patients. These aspects of patient care are essential to the patient's well-being and are integral components in providing quality care. But they do not constitute skilled services under the Medicare program and are not reimbursable unless provided in conjunction with a covered skilled service.

Skilled care has three components that distinguish it from

unskilled care, which does not require professional health training. One component is the observation and/or assessment of the patient. The patient's condition is such that the reasonable probability exists that significant changes may occur that would require the skills of a professional to evaluate the need for modification of the plan of treatment. It is considered medically reasonable and necessary for a professional to supplement the physician's personal contact with the patient; however, only the physician may order needed changes in the plan of treatment.

Another component is the giving of direct skilled services to a patient when the ability to provide such services requires the knowledge, skills, and judgement of a professional.

A third component, the one we are concerned with in this text, is the teaching of the patient and/or caregiver to carry out the appropriate services and observations. In addition to the requirement of an intermittent skilled need, the beneficiary must also be under the care of a physician and confined to his or her home.

## Intermittent Skilled Care

"Intermittent" is defined in Section 204.1 of HIM-11. In order for the patient to meet the intermittent requirement, he must have a medically predictable recurring need for skilled care at least once every 60 days. There are certain exceptions to the 60-day limitation:

- a *silicone* catheter change that is required only at 90-day intervals
- manual fecal disimpaction that is likely to recur but is impossible to predict
- skilled observation for changes in the level of care at 90-day intervals for a blind diabetic patient who self-injects insulin.

Another exception to the intermittent requirement is when a patient expires or is institutionalized after the first skilled visit and the home health agency had no way of knowing this would occur. In this instance, the one visit would be reimbursable; however, a one-time visit to give an injection, draw blood for laboratory studies, or make a skilled observation and report to the physician would not be considered intermittent because its recurrence is not medically predictable.

Daily visits are also an exception to the intermittent requirement and are coverable if justified in writing by the patient's attending physician indicating the medical necessity for the visits and expected period of time they will be needed. Daily visits as defined by the Health Care Financing Administration (HCFA) may be 5, 6, or 7 days per week, depending on the particular fiscal intermediary's definition.

It has been our experience with fiscal intermediaries in HCFA Region VI that "daily visits" was interpreted to mean 7 days per week. We have dealt with denials of reimbursement because the patient was not seen on Saturday and Sunday. The fiscal intermediary's rational was: if the patient and/or caregiver did not need skilled intervention on the weekend, was it necessary to see them 5 days per week? This could have been avoided by specific documentation of the situation. For example, the daughter was an R.N. but lived 200 miles away and was home with her mother only on infrequent weekends.

Due to the increase in home care since the inception of the prospective payment system (PPS) and advances in medical technology for the delivery of high-tech care in the home, e.g., mechanical ventilation, infusion therapy, multiple visits in a 24-hour period have become necessary. These multiple visits are reimbursable if they are reasonable and necessary and are not for an extended period of time. If the patient's needs could be met more effectively and safely in an institutional setting, the visits would probably be denied. These types of cases are usually referred to Level III of the medical review process for a claim determination.

In May 1984, HCFA issued a policy statement that clarified the definition of "intermittent," but it is an issue that is still not completely resolved. Home care standards of practice are changing more rapidly than the government programs that regulate the Medicare-certified home health agencies. As home health care providers, we must stay in tune with the changes and become active leaders in the local, state, and national organizations concerned with improving the standards of practice in home care; increasing the awareness of legislators, both local and federal, of issues that need to be assessed and resolved in home care; and educating the general public concerning services available in their home.

## Homebound Status

As mentioned previously, the patient must be confined to his home, i.e., homebound, to qualify for home health benefits under the Medicare program. Homebound requirements are found in HIM-11, Section 208.4 and as a cross reference in more detail in

*Medicare Intermediary Manual, Part 3: Claims Process* (HCFA Publication no. 13-3).

The following is an overview of the homebound criteria found in these references:

- physician certifies that the patient is confined to his home
- patient's medical condition restricts his ability to leave home without the aid of a supportive device, special transportation, or the assistance of another person
- absence from home requires a considerable and taxing effort
- absences from home are infrequent and for a short period of time
- absences from home are to receive medical treatment
- absences from home do not indicate the patient is able to seek medical treatment outside the home.

Be aware that these criteria may be interpreted differently by your fiscal intermediary. It is the nurse's responsibility to understand the homebound criteria and apply them judiciously to each patient qualifying with functional limitations. The patient's diagnosis or condition may not be enough to qualify for the homebound criteria, e.g., diabetes mellitus, cardiac condition, cancer.

## WHAT CONSTITUTES A SKILLED TEACHING VISIT

Under the Medicare program, the home health benefit reimburses only for intermittent skilled services required during the acute and subacute phases of an illness or injury. Once the patient's condition stabilizes, services are no longer reimbursable.

Skilled teaching of a responsible adult to irrigate a catheter, prepare and follow a therapeutic diet, carry out therapeutic exercises, administer injections, if appropriate, and be aware of signs and symptoms that should be reported to the physician can be initiated during the acute or subacute phase of illness. The patient's care may be continued when the skilled services of observation and evaluation or direct skilled care are no longer required. Therefore, to teach the patient self-care (and/or instruct the caregiver in the care of the patient) is one of the most important skilled services provided as a home care benefit, as it greatly contributes to the goals of recovery and rehabilitation.

There are several factors used by Medicare to determine if a teaching visit constitutes a skilled service, the foremost being whether or not the teaching provided requires the skills and knowledge of a professional (or if the teaching could be provided by the average nonmedical person). For example, the patient who has edema in his lower extremities and is instructed by the nurse to elevate his feet would not qualify because the average nonmedical person possesses enough knowledge to instruct the patient to elevate his feet.

Even though a skilled procedure is taught to the patient or caregiver, the procedure or service can still be performed by the home health care professional as a skilled service.[1] For example, for instruction in self-irrigation of a colostomy, both the teaching and performance of the service are considered skilled; therefore, when the patient has mastered the procedure, he is functioning as a skilled person. However, if the patient is unable to or physically or mentally incapable of learning the procedure being taught, and there is no one else available or willing to be taught, the performance of the procedure will continue to be considered a skilled service if performed by the nurse.[2]

On the other hand, a service is not considered a skilled service simply because it is performed by or under the direct supervision of a licensed nurse or therapist. When the nature of a service is such that it can safely and adequately be self-administered or performed by the average nonmedical person without the direct supervision of a licensed nurse or therapist, it is an unskilled service without regard to who performs it. However, if the nurse provides personal care to a bedridden patient while teaching the caregiver how to care for him, this service would be considered skilled during the teaching phase because the knowledge of a professional is required to instruct in the care of a bedridden patient. On the other hand, even if no one was available or willing to learn to provide personal care, it would not constitute a skilled service even though it was performed by a nurse.[3]

## TEACHING AND TRAINING ACTIVITIES THAT MEDICARE CONSIDERS REIMBURSABLE

HIM-11 lists twelve examples of teaching and training activities that are considered to require the skills or knowledge of a nurse or therapist, thus constituting a skilled service.[4] These twelve examples are incorporated in the following list:

1. Give an injection, e.g., insulin, B12, certain antibiotics.
2. Irrigate a catheter, e.g., Foley, suprapubic, subclavian, Hickman.
3. Care for a colostomy, ileostomy, or gastrostomy.

4. Administer medical gases.
5. Prepare and follow a therapeutic diet.
6. Apply dressings to wounds involving prescription medications and aseptic techniques.
7. Carry out bladder training.
8. Carry out bowel training for incontinence *only*.
9. Perform self-care activities of daily living (dressing, eating, personal hygiene, etc.) through use of special techniques and adaptive devices when he has suffered a loss of function.
10. Align and position a bedbound patient.
11. Perform transfer activities, e.g., from bed to bed, bed to chair or wheelchair, wheelchair to bathtub or toilet.
12. Ambulate by means of crutches, walker, cane, etc.
13. Engage in therapeutic exercises when he has suffered a loss of function.
14. Care for a bedridden patient.
15. Care for an intravenous (IV) site.[5]

This is not an inclusive list; any teaching or training activity to be provided must be evaluated to determine if it constitutes a skilled service.

Through years of experience as Medicare-certified home health care providers, we have identified the following general criteria as tests that Medicare may use to determine coverage. The following questions can help you make this determination:

• Are the skills or knowledge of a professional nurse or therapist needed to accomplish the teaching?
• Are the teaching visits reasonable and necessary?
• Is the teaching pertinent to the active treatment of the patient's illness or disability?

Another important consideration involves the duplication of services by different disciplines seeing the same patient. For example, if a patient requires the skills of a nurse and therapist, each discipline must use its *unique* skill to instruct the patient in his care. This becomes crucial in the area of therapeutic exercises and activities of daily living. The patient may be receiving the services of a registered nurse, home health aide, physical therapist, and occupational therapist. It is of utmost importance that the patient's condition warrant the *unique* skills of the physical therapist and occupational therapist to carry out the physician's plan of treatment safely and effectively; otherwise Medicare may determine that these services could be carried out by the licensed nurse or, in some instances, performed safely and effectively by the home health aide. This determination could result in a denial of reimbursement for the physical therapy and occupational therapy services.

There are no hard and fast rules establishing a particular exercise program that would require the skills of a licensed nurse, physical therapist, or occupational therapist. Therefore, the responsibility falls upon the professional to document the patient's condition, indicating the degree of sensory perception, motor deficits, and loss of function. Proper documentation enables Medicare to make an accurate determination of the services covered.

As one of the major components of skilled care identified in the Medicare guidelines, teaching can be the only skilled service provided, but the need for teaching must be readily evident and requires in depth documentation.

## THE REASONABLE AND NECESSARY ASPECT OF PATIENT TEACHING

Teaching visits are subject to the test of reasonableness and necessity as outlined in HIM-11, Section 204.3. Reimbursement may be made for skilled nursing services required by an individual only if such services are found to be reasonable and necessary to the treatment of the individual's illness or injury. To be considered reasonable and necessary for the treatment of an illness or injury, the services furnished must be consistent with the nature and severity of the individual's illness or injury, his particular medical needs, and the accepted standards of medical practice.[6]

Among the factors Medicare uses to determine if a teaching visit is reasonable or necessary are

- the date of onset of the patient's illness or injury
- the length of stay in an institution, i.e., hospital, skilled nursing facility, or rehabilitation unit
- the length of service with the home health agency
- previous admissions to the home health agency for the same illness or injury
- physician's order for the teaching and training activities
- the consistency of the teaching and training activities with the nature and severity of the individual's illness or injury
- the learning ability of the patient's family member or caregiver being taught
- previous services from another home health agency

- mental status of the person to whom teaching is directed
- literacy level of the person to whom the teaching is directed
- patient compliance (indicate if noncompliance is due to a knowledge deficit or to patient will).

Teaching should never be initiated without first obtaining a physician's order. The order should be pertinent to and consistent with the patient's illness or injury. Teaching is an accepted nursing function and a vital part of good nursing practice, but in home health the physician must coordinate all care rendered, and therefore an order must be obtained.

Ensuring that the teaching and training activities are consistent with the patient's illness or injury is the first test in determining if the service is reasonable and necessary. This should be a part of your initial and ongoing evaluation process during the patient's entire length of service.

The date of onset is also very important to Medicare in making the determination of reasonableness and/or necessity. An example would be a patient who was diagnosed as a Type II diabetic 15 years ago, has been maintained by diet and oral hypoglycemics, recently experienced an acute exacerbation of the disease, and was placed on insulin injections daily. It would not be reasonable or necessary to continue home health visits after the patient mastered self-administration of the insulin injections just to instruct in an American Diabetic Association (ADA) diet of which the patient had a good understanding and to which he had adhered for 15 years. Consideration must also be given to whether the teaching provided in the home is reinforcement of teaching begun in the hospital, skilled nursing facility, or rehabilitation unit during a previous home health admission or is the initial instruction received by the patient for the particular illness or injury.

For reinforcement of previous teaching or training, fewer visits would generally be required and allowed than for initial training. For example, for a patient who had a cataract extraction and was seen by home health professionals postoperatively, visits to instruct him concerning signs and symptoms of complications to be aware of, dressings changes, etc. would not be covered for a second extraction since it would be expected that all teaching activities were completed during the previous admission for this illness. This would be true even if the patient was seen during the second admission by a different home health agency.

If the patient, family member, or caregiver being instructed has a learning deficit, poor comprehension, a condition that impedes memory, or is illiterate, the home health agency must document the need for additional visits. Although additional visits may be allowed in these circumstances, they cannot be allowed beyond the point where it would be appropriate to conclude that the individual cannot be taught to perform the required service.

For example, for a Type II diabetic patient who is placed on an 1,800 calorie ADA diet but shows poor comprehension and is a slow learner, additional visits might be allowed if these circumstances were included in the documentation of the patient's educational assessment, teaching plan, and visit record. Conversely, if the patient experienced intermittent memory loss or confusion and could not remember what had been taught during the previous visit, additional visits to instruct him would probably not be allowed since it would be doubtful he would benefit from additional instruction. In situations of this nature, a responsible family member or caregiver should receive the instruction.

Patient compliance must also be a consideration. The licensed nurse or therapist must assess and evaluate the reason for noncompliance. If noncompliance is due to will rather than lack of knowledge, it may be reasonably expected that the patient will not comply with the instructions, and the teaching and training activities should be discontinued if all avenues of teaching have been investigated and implemented and have failed. If teaching was the only reason this patient was on service, then visits should also be discontinued.

It has been our experience that length of service is very easy for Medicare to identify for any claim submitted. A claim submitted with teaching as the main skilled service provided with a length of service of more than 90 days will be reviewed carefully by the medical review department. We cannot emphasize enough the importance of documentation in these instances. If you have been instructing a patient for 60 days or longer, you must re-evaluate your teaching and his comprehension level and progress and determine in your professional judgement how much longer he will need the instructions of a licensed nurse or therapist. Your documentation should reflect this evaluation and your plans concerning the patient's specific need.

---

**REFERENCES**

1. U.S. Department of Health and Human Services, "Coverage of Home Health Services," in *Home Health Agency Manual*, Publication no.11, Section 204.2C (Washington, DC:

Health Care Financing Administration, 1983), p. 14.3.
2. Ibid.
3. Ibid., Section 204.2B, p. 14.3.
4. Ibid., Section 204.4B, p. 14.5.
5. Ibid.
6. Ibid., Section 204.3, p. 14.4.

**BIBLIOGRAPHY**

McHatton, M. "A Theory for Timely Teaching." *American Journal of Nursing* 85, no. 7 (July 1985):797-800.
Miller, A. "When Is the Time Ripe for Teaching?" *American Journal of Nursing* 85, no. 7 (July 1985):801-804.
*Patient Teaching: Nurses' Reference Library.* Springhouse, Penn.: Springhouse Corp., 1987.
Spiegel, A.D. *Home Healthcare.* Owings Mill, Md.: National Health Publishing, 1983.

# Home Care Strictly by the Rules

*Diane J. Omdahl*

Whether you're playing Monopoly or crossing the street, you need to know the rules. And so does the home care nurse when dealing with Medicare.

You'll find the rules governing the delivery of home care services in the Medicare Home Health Agency Manual, Publication 11 of the Health Care Financing Administration (HCFA), commonly referred to as HIM 11. Designed to guide your care delivery and documentation, the rules form the foundation of the Medicare home care program. But because the rules are far from complete and less than explicit about what is and isn't covered, we're forced to interpret them when we care for patients covered by Medicare.

## ROUTINE ASSESSMENT

Let's apply the rules to everyday practice in a skilled nursing service. Section 204.4A of the Manual defines "observation and evaluation" as follows:

*Where a physician concludes that a patient's condition is such that the reasonable probability exists that significant changes may occur which would require his or her skills or the skills of the licensed nurse to evaluate the need for modification in the plan of treatment or to consider institutionalization, it would be appropriate for the physician to request a nurse to supplement his or her personal contacts with the patient.*

Looking past the ten verbs in that statement, you'll see several key phrases that affect your care delivery and documentation:

*Reasonable probability exists that significant changes may occur.*
You must know why you are evaluating the patient's condition and
what problems may develop. Show the need for assessment by
documenting the patient's prior instability in your initial assessment
and in your nursing history. For example, if the patient has
congestive heart failure, it is reasonably probable that he could
develop fluid retention - a significant change - again.

*Requires the skills of the licensed nurse.* Your actions must be
appropriate and be based on your professional knowledge and
expertise. For that same patient, you'd monitor his weight, activity,
and breathlessness; check for pedal edema; and evaluate his
sodium intake - all appropriate and skilled actions to check for
fluid retention.

*Need for modification in the plan of treatment.* If you detect fluid
retention, you'd notify the physician who would modify the plan
accordingly.

*Physician concludes* and *appropriate for the physician to request
the nurse to supplement his contacts.* HCFA and its intermediaries
can deny reimbursement for evaluation if they find no evidence of
a physician's involvement, even though evaluating a patient is well
within the scope of nursing licensure. Document your discussion
with the physician as well as any changes in plan clearly, then have
the physician countersign your statement.

## THE LETTER OF THE LAW

Suppose a patient receives daily skilled nursing visits for six
weeks. The intermediary denies payment for care after the third
week because the visits were not medically reasonable. You check
the Manual, Section 204.1 to see why. Here's what the rules say
about a patient whose prognosis warrants daily visits beyond three
weeks:

*As soon as the patient's physician makes this judgement [to extend
nursing visits] which should usually be made before the end of the
three-week period, the home health agency must forward medical
documentation justifying the need for additional services.*

You could have prevented the denial by having the physician
prescribe visits for three weeks, at first, then, near the end of the
third week, by having him prescribe the additional visits, and
submitting the documentation. Yes, it's extra paperwork and
aggravation, but with rules as specific as these, we have few
options.

## APPEALING HCFA'S DENIALS

Just as we have to interpret the rules when actually delivering care, so too do HCFA and its intermediaries when making decisions about payment. In 1986 and 1987, HCFA instructed its intermediaries to consider care delivered five, six, or seven times a week daily care.[1] Even though we disagreed with that interpretation, we had to live by it.

So what's the use of knowing the rules if they're subject to such broad interpretation? One good reason is that HCFA's interpretations are not always correct. In 1988, a judge ruled that HCFA's definition of daily care was improper.[2] Here's another case in point.

Section 208.4 of the Manual defines homebound as follows:

*An individual does not have to be confined to his bed to be considered confined to his home.*

Over the years, HCFA has so tightened the criteria that some patients have been denied service on the grounds that they cannot be considered homebound if they can get out of bed. As more and more claims were denied, Congress stepped in with the Omnibus Reconciliation Act of 1987. The Act clarified the definition of homebound as follows:

*While an individual does not have to be bedridden to be confined to his home, the condition must be such that there exists a normal inability to leave home.*

Of course we cannot always rely on an act of Congress to uphold the original rules, so we must appeal denials through established channels. The appeal process is lengthy, but often appeals are successful. The National Association for Home Care reports reversal rates of 20 to 25 percent at the reconsideration level and administrative law judge (ALJ) reversal rates averaging 60 percent nationwide.[3] And some agencies report ALJ reversal rates of 90 to 95 percent.[3] When you support your interpretations with the rules and show how they apply to your patient, you build a strong foundation for appeal.

## SAY WHAT YOU MEAN

An agency admits a postop cataract patient to service. The original plan specifies two visits for postcataract evaluation and teaching. On the second visit, the patient's blood pressure skyrockets. The physician orders more visits - for evaluating the patient and for teaching him to take another drug and to modify his diet. The agency documents the change in circumstances and the physician contact.  Initially denied, the additional visits are declared reimbursable on appeal because the agency had followed the rules, as in Section 204.4:

*However, should complicating secondary conditions be present or develop, additional visits may be reimbursable upon appropriate documentation.*

Finally, knowing the rules will help you strengthen your case for the delivery of other services.  For example, Sections 205.1B, 205.2B, and 205.3B, addressing physical, speech, and occupational therapy, state:

*There must be an expectation that the patient's condition will improve significantly in a reasonable and generally predictable period of time.*

Validate the patient's need for therapy and restorative potential in your initial assessment, therefore, by documenting the patient's pre-accident or pre-injury level of performance.  If the patient was a dance instructor before she fractured her hip, for example, document that you expect she will improve significantly in a reasonable period of time.  The therapy plan must incorporate clear and measurable goals that can be achieved by a specific time.

Or, for medical social services, consider the rules in Section 206.1:

*Medical social services must be needed because social problems (economic, marital, environmental, etc.) exist which are or will be an impediment to the effective treatment of the patient's medical condition or rate of recovery.*

If the patient is so wrapped up in financial worries that he cannot pay attention to your teaching, document that fact, spelling out the connection clearly.  Or, if the patient is not following the treatment plan because he wants to retaliate against his wife, note the details and the reason as the patient states it.  ("Weight gain of five pounds in three days.  States he quit taking the diuretic because his wife doesn't care what happens to him anyway.")

Once you get the knack of precisely documenting the situation to fit the rules, you're on the way to improving reimbursement for the services your patients need.

---

**REFERENCES**

1. Memorandum from Robert A. Streimer to Mary Townsend, November 11, 1986.
2. NAHC wins major lawsuit. *NAHC Report* 273A, Aug 5, 1988.
3. Cabin, W. D. Using a spreadsheet to manage claim denial activity. *Home Health Line* 13:39, Feb 8, 1988.

# The Denial Dilemma

*Marilyn Harris, RN, MSN, CNAA*

A home health agency's administration and board of directors have just issued the following:

## Proclamation

**WHEREAS:** A patient has been referred to this home health agency for care of a small decubitus ulcer;

**WHEREAS:** The patient has health insurance through the Medicare program;

**WHEREAS:** The patient and physician have requested that nursing care be billed to Medicare;

**WHEREAS:** A small decubitus ulcer does not meet the Medicare requirement for a skilled nursing visit (Section 204.4, J2);

**WHEREAS:** Reimbursement is important for the survival of this agency;

**THEREFORE:** Be it resolved that the patient's admission to the home health agency be delayed until the "small" decubitus ulcer becomes "large" so that nursing care for the nursing diagnosis of *Actual Alteration in Skin Integrity* can be billed to Medicare.

Be it further resolved, and known to all involved, that payment for this skilled nursing service may not be forthcoming due to a technical or medical denial.

Be it further resolved that such denial will be reviewed by supervisory and administrative staff and appropriate reopening, reconsideration, or other necessary action initiated.

The home health nurse's first reaction to this proclamation would probably be: "That's absurd! The patient needs quality nursing care now, including teaching the family how to prevent further deterioration of the small ulcer. The decubitus should not be allowed to deteriorate." I agree! But across the country home health care nurses are having to confront the vast difference between identified patient needs and the important role of professional nursing interventions in meeting these needs on the one hand, and the lack of reimbursement for these services on the other hand.

Visit any home health agency in the United States or attend a regional, state, or national meeting and you can hear and feel the frustration, anger, disappointment, and low morale at all staff levels because of the increasing number of medical and technical denials for Medicare services, reductions in the allowable length of home health care due to more rigid interpretations and regulations, more frequent re-hospitalizations, and the resulting concerns for fiscal stability.

Many health care issues are being raised today: "Do the current reimbursement stipulations allow for the provision of quality care?" "Are patients ready for discharge when they are discharged from service (that is, are they independent in their treatments and knowledgeable about their medications)?" "Are nurses and other health care workers able to provide needed services to the extent indicated by the patient's condition?"

The major reason for the existence of most home health agencies is to provide quality health care services to those individuals who need these services. But home health care costs money and agencies must be financially sound in order to continue to provide services. During the past months Medicare denials have had a significant impact on the solvency of an increasing number of agencies.

I believe that home care nurses are special individuals. Besides providing professional services in less than ideal settings, these nurses must be able to cope with all types of everyday problems, such as dogs, cats, insects, bad weather, poor road conditions, and various potential hazards. On top of all this, the federal government, through its fiscal intermediary (FI), expects nurses to be superhuman! For example, all Plan of Treatment forms must be completed correctly and in detail in order to avoid a denial of payment. The FI does not know that a nurse may have made a late night emergency visit and written out a verbal order to cover the extra visit, but that she had no opportunity to write the order on Form 485 before it was sent out with the bill the following day. Such a visit will undoubtedly be denied for this patient! The explanation for the next denial will be just as "logical."

The nurse is expected to chart perfectly - from both a technical and medical viewpoint - while also maintaining the agency's productivity standard (which is necessary for fiscal survival). Meanwhile, the nurse is also providing quality, comprehensive care to a patient and family who may be totally confused when they receive a letter advising them that the nursing care they have been given is "unreasonable" or that they are not "homebound." Is it any wonder that the typical home health care agency's management and staff are frustrated and concerned about patient care and agency liability?

There are no easy answers; in this column, I am simply raising questions and issues that are common to home health care nurses. I invite you to write in and share your own experiences and solutions to specific problems you have encountered. How do you document the need for nursing care of small or large decubitus ulcers? Do you take photographs when the patient is admitted to service, and then document progress or the lack of it with this visual tool? Has this approach been successful? I, as well as the other readers of *Home Healthcare Nurse*, look forward to your solutions to the current denial dilemma. Why not write your own proclamation!

―――――――――――――――――――――*CHAPTER 2*

# Skilled Documentation

# Charting that Makes it through the Medicare Maze

*Helen M. Magliozzi, RN, BSN*

Published in *RN* June 1990.

John Stone, a 92-year-old diabetic just discharged from the hospital, needs daily insulin injections and wound care for severe leg ulcers. A home care nurse begins visiting him every afternoon. But when her agency seeks Medicare reimbursement, the claim is denied. The reason? Documentation submitted with the claim states that Mr. Stone "leaves the house" for bi-weekly whirlpool treatments. The Medicare claims examiner interpreted those words to mean that Mr. Stone isn't homebound and is therefore ineligible for home care coverage.

A recent update in Medicare's home health manual and a clarification of its provisions have reduced the incidence of such senseless denials, but your documentation is still crucial. Charting that focuses on what's wrong with the patient, the likelihood of any complications, and the reason he requires continuing home care is the key to claims' approval.

As quality assurance coordinator, I review our nurses' notes to make sure they do just that. Knowing what I look for can help you chart in a way most likely to result in Medicare reimbursement. Since other third-party payers frequently follow Medicare's lead, it will help you be an advocate for all your home care patients.

## ELIGIBILITY DEPENDS ON HOMEBOUND STATUS

Medicare will reimburse for home care only if the patient is homebound. The Medicare manual defines that as a "normal inability to leave home," or being so weak or feeble that leaving home would require "a considerable taxing effort."

Patients who have limited mobility, whether because they depend on crutches or other assistive devices or because they're blind, senile, or otherwise unable to go out unassisted, are considered to be homebound. So are patients with posthospital weakness whose activities have been restricted by their physician. Medicare now even acknowledges that a patient who's homebound may leave the house for medical care, like hemodialysis, whirlpool treatments, or adult day care, that meets medical needs -- provided the outside care doesn't duplicate skilled services provided at home.

To ensure coverage, document the reason your patient is homebound. After each visit, document it again. Use measurable, objective criteria when possible: "Patient short of breath after walking 20 feet," for instance, is better than "limited endurance." Documenting that Mr. Stone was "taken to sterile whirlpool treatments" would've been more specific than saying he "leaves the house." No doubt his care would have been reimbursed.

## POSTHOSPITAL CARE AND THE THREE-WEEK RULE

In the past, Medicare routinely denied payment for home care provided to guard against posthospital complications if those problems didn't develop. Presently, home care is reimbursable for three weeks after discharge as long as there's a reasonable possibility that serious complications *could* develop, whether they do or not. Care will be reimbursable, then, if you document potential problems and explain how they're linked to the patient's primary condition.

Start by identifying the problem: "Patient having trouble following a low-sodium diet," you might write about a patient with newly diagnosed CHF. Add that failure to change her eating patterns puts her at risk for fluid overload. Do *not* write or imply that the care you're providing is preventive: if you do, Medicare won't pay.

Documenting a case when care stretches beyond three weeks is a balancing act: If you report no progress, Medicare is apt to discontinue reimbursement, claiming that home care has not been and will not be successful and that the condition is chronic. If you report too much progress, however, Medicare may simply conclude home care is no longer needed.

Go for a happy medium, showing some improvement but emphasizing that far more skilled care is needed. "Patient has learned to draw up insulin and test glucose independently," you might write about a diabetic who's just become dependent on insulin, "but still requires instruction in self-injection and diet."

## HOW TO DEFINE AND DOCUMENT SKILLED CARE

A task that must be performed by an RN or done under the supervision of an RN is considered to be skilled care, according to Medicare, as long as it's reasonable and necessary. That, of course, depends on the patient's condition.

A task isn't considered skilled care just because a nurse performs it, though, and it doesn't stop being classified as skilled care because a member of the family or some other caregiver has been taught how to carry it out.

Observation and assessment, teaching, case management, and administering meds IV, IM, or subcutaneously are considered skilled care. Tube feeding, nasopharyngeal and trach aspiration, venipuncture, and wound, catheter, and ostomy care are other examples.

Some interventions qualify under some circumstances but not under others. Vitamin $B_{12}$ injections, for instance, are reimbursable if given to treat pernicious anemia but not if used to treat generalized posthospital weakness.

Undoubtedly you give skilled care at each visit. The trick is to identify it properly, link it to the patient's primary diagnosis, and explain why it's reasonable and necessary.

Again, be as objective and specific as possible. For wound care, chart the size of the wound and the amount of drainage at every visit. If a patient on home IV antibiotic therapy was taught to administer the antibiotic himself while in the hospital, explain that he needs help at home handling the medication, starting the infusion, flushing the line, and assessing the antibiotic's effectiveness.

It's fine to use a word like "reinstruct" to describe what you're doing. Avoid words that suggest that nothing has changed, such as reinforce, monitor, chronic, and stable.

## ANCILLARY SERVICES AND CASE MANAGEMENT

Medicare recently added case management — by an RN or physical therapist — to its list of what constitutes skilled care. The nurse/case manager may oversee the care of a patient whose complex needs call for unskilled services such as a homemaker, a home health aide, or Meals on Wheels. The nurse must visit the patient at least once every 60 days for re-evaluation.

If the unskilled services and your services as case manager are still necessary — if, in fact, they're keeping the patient out of the hospital — your documentation should explain why. Chart problems and potential problems, including safety and functional limitations and the complexity of the patient's condition.

But aim for balance. Medicare will not pay for these services or for case management indefinitely, so it's important to identify short- and long-term goals and show progress in achieving them. "Patient maintains adequate nutrition," might be the short-term goal for a patient getting Meals on Wheels. The long-term goal: "Patient is able to remain at home without RN supervision," which could happen only after his nutritional status stabilized.

There's no need for an RN case manager when only skilled ancillary services like PT, OT, or social work, are required. A doctor must order physical or occupational therapy, so you don't have to document need. To justify a social worker's visits, documentation should show that social or emotional problems are interfering with the care plan — for instance, depression causing anorexia in one whose recovery depends on a well-balanced diet.

Documenting with reimbursement in mind takes practice. If you realize the words you use can mean the difference between approval and denial, I'm sure you'll see it's worth the effort.

# Home Care Charting Dos and Don'ts

*Diane J. Omdahl*

Mr. Jones, age 79, had a cholecystectomy and developed a postoperative wound dehiscence and infection. He had had insulin-dependent diabetes for nine years and had a history of congestive heart failure. Recently discharged from the hospital, he lives with his 69-year-old wife in a two-story home.

The nurse visited the patient daily after hospital discharge. On the eighth day, she documented her visit as follows:

"Mr. Jones is up ad lib. Wife knows dressing-change procedure and can describe clean technique. Abdominal wound healing.

"Patient able to administer insulin with good technique. Reviewed 1,200-calorie ADA diet with wife. 1+ pedal edema noted in left lower extremity. Will observe. Dr. Samuels called. No changes in medications. Patient on Lasix 40 mg for two years."

As written, the nurse's documentation may not have justified the six further visits she planned. Although Mr. Jones needed care, the documentation was incomplete and misleading. Reimbursement by Medicare may not have been forthcoming.

The following review shows how the nurse's recording can be improved to reflect not only the skilled care that she actually did but why continued intervention was necessary. Each phrase is followed by the literal interpretation the fiscal intermediary might use, then by the actual facts, and finally by suggestions to improve documentation.

### Up ad lib.

*Fiscal intermediary's (FI) interpretation:* If the patient is up as desired, he is not home bound.

*Facts:* Mr. Jones was up as he desired, but he experienced cramping abdominal pain and pulling with diaphoresis and faintness when he walked. He could not walk more than 25 feet. Such pain and discomfort severely restricted his ability to leave his home.

*What's needed:* Describe the facts in detail. This example shows the danger of summarizing.

### Wife knows dressing change procedure.

*FI's interpretation:* If the wife knows the procedure, she can change the dressings. No visits are needed.

*Facts:* The wife could recount the steps in the wound care and dressing-care procedure; however, she could not look at the wound. With the nurse's help, the wife was working to overcome her fear and perform the procedure.

*What's needed:* Include all the facts. Because the wife knew what to do did not mean she could do it.

### Able to describe clean technique.

*FI's interpretation:* If the wife knows clean technique, there is no further need for teaching.

*Facts:* The wife could describe clean technique but she could not carry it out. The home was very unclean. The nurse was assisting the wife in a plan to clean the home to make the technique possible.

*What's needed:* Describe the home and the wife's limited performance.

### Abdominal wound healing.

*FI's interpretation:* Future visits may be denied as not medically necessary if the wound is healing.

*Facts:* On admission, the wound measured 9 cm by 4 cm and was 2 cm deep. There was a copious amount of purulent drainage. By the eighth day, the wound measured 7 cm by 2 cm by 0.5 cm. Drainage was less and was serosanguineous.

*What's needed:* The wound was improving but not healed. Describe the dimensions, drainage, and appearance and let the facts show the degree of healing.

### Patient able to administer own insulin with good technique.

*FI's interpretation:* Because the patient has been on insulin several years and demonstrates good technique, no teaching is needed in this area.

*Facts:* Although the patient could give himself insulin, he misread the syringe calibrations. The nurse had to teach the patient how to read the syringe and how to draw up the correct amount.

*What's needed:* Include new findings (patient's impaired vision) that affect the patient's performance and demonstrate the need for teaching.

### Reviewed the 1,200-calorie ADA diet with wife.

*FI's interpretation:* Repetition or review of teaching is not reimbursable.

*Facts:* Until he was hospitalized, Mr. Jones had been on a 2,000-calorie ADA diet. The physician ordered a change in diet because the patient was overweight. The wife did not know how to make the necessary changes.

*What's needed:* Note changes that justify the intervention. Do not use words, such as "reviewed" or "reinforced," that imply the patient or wife already know the information.

### 1+ pedal edema noted in left lower extremity. Dr. Samuels called. No changes in medications. Will observe.

*FI's interpretation:* If there are no changes anticipated in the plan of treatment, then observation and evaluation may not be reimbursed.

*Facts:* MD did not change the medication but he did ask the nurse to monitor the edema closely and inform him of any changes. He also wanted the nurse to assess the patient's diet for sodium.

*What's needed:* Spell out the MD's instructions, even if there are no medication changes. Your continued observations may lead to changes in the treatment plan.

### The patient has been on Lasix 40 mg for two years.

*FI's interpretation:* Since the patient has been on furosemide (Lasix) for two years, it appears that the edema is a chronic problem related to the patient's CHF. Skilled intervention for a chronic problem is not reimbursed.

*Facts:* Mr. Jones has never had lower-extremity edema. This is a new problem that requires skilled intervention.

*What's needed:* Again state the facts (no history of pedal edema) and other skilled interventions (elevating legs, limiting sodium intake). You do not have to mention furosemide here as it is included in locator 13 on the HCFA 485 form. The nurse also did not record any skilled interventions.

The nurse had reviewed the records of the patient's blood and urine testing, insulin administration, and food intake.   She monitored the patient's temperature and vital signs, cardiopulmonary status, fluid intake, and urinary and bowel functions. Such observation and evaluation would detect problems that might be anticipated after surgery.

The nurse also taught the patient palliative measures to control the edema, such as elevating his legs when seated. she taught him how to ease the pain during walking, such as using a pillow as a splint. The nurse also changed the dressing, a skilled procedure.

An example of documentation that would more accurately reflect the skilled interventions would be: BP, 138/76; T, 98.6; P, 76; R, 22; Lungs clear   Mr. Jones is only walking three to four times a day.  At these times, he experiences pulling abdominal pain with diaphoresis and faintness and must sit down after walking 20 to 25 feet. Taught to use a pillow to splint the wound. Also taught that frequent walking is necessary to prevent complications of inactivity. Patient says he will try to walk a little every hour.

Wife able to recite exact dressing-change procedure but still experiences nausea when she thinks about looking at the wound. Small amount of dried serosanguineous drainage on dressing. Wound cleansed with 1:1 solution $H_2O_2$ and $H_2O$.   Wound measures 7×2×0.5 cm.

Wife did look at the wound briefly without nausea.   Wife reports she cleaned the bedroom.  Rests of home remains dirty and unkempt.  Wife says she will begin cleaning kitchen today.

Urine test results negative. FBS this morning was 120.

Patient demonstrated ability to draw up exact amount of insulin today. He still is unsure of syringe calibrations and asked nurse to verify dose. He demonstrated correct administration technique.

Wife asked for a review of the meal plan she has developed. She still uses more fruit and bread exchanges than the 1,200-calorie ADA diet permits.   Meal plan corrected and wife instructed in use of fruit exchanges.

1+ pedal edema noted in left lower extremity. Patient states he "has never had swelling before" and has been taking his Lasix every day.

Called Dr. Samuels.  He wants edema observed and sodium intake assessed.  MD also wants to be informed of increase in edema.  Mr. Jones instructed to elevate legs and to write down all food consumed for the next 24 hours.*

\* This example is long but demonstrates the content that should be included in the record to justify Medicare service. Besides the visit note, you can use the care plan, learning programs, wound care checklist, and other supplementary forms to document services.

# Visit Notes

*Pat Carr, RN*

"Patients come and patients go, but a visit note lasts forever."

For the nursing staff of a home health agency, a visit note may also take forever. Forever to be written by the field nurse, forever to be processed by the supervisor, and forever to be reconciled with all the other notes in the chart by the chart auditor.

There is nothing more basic to home health than the skilled nursing visit. The visit note is simply a written record of that event. It does not need to be elaborate, but it does need to be lucid and understandable. It does not need to be a work of literary art, but it does need to be readable. The visit note must accurately reflect what took place during the nursing visit and it must be consistent with the other visit notes written for the individual patient.

Accuracy and consistency can be achieved, no matter how many nurses see a particular patient and no matter how complex that patient's case is. What is needed is a mental blueprint. If each nurse keeps that blueprint in mind, accuracy and consistency in charting will naturally follow.

Start with objective observations. Assess the patient, keeping in mind the diagnosis and current treatment. Begin the note with a concise and detailed description of physical findings pertinent to the patient's problem. Measure anything that is measurable. Remember, a centimeter is the same size regardless of who holds the ruler. Assess drainage on dressings in terms that say something. "Dime-sized amount thick opaque yellow drainage on old dressing" is more meaningful than "Scant purulent drainage." Assessments of other objective data should be equally clear. "Few rales heard right lower lobe" says something definite, and pinpoints an area to be assessed on the next visit. "Scattered rales" gives no definite information, and leaves the next nurse in the home with no point of comparison.

Objective data should not be charted in a way that leaves the documentation open to interpretation. This does not need to mean longer, more involved notes. What is needed is a few minutes' thought about the difference between subjective and objective. "Denies constipation" is a subjective statement. "BM yesterday" covers the same ground, and is clear and objective. Describing a patient's activity level as "limited" is subjective. "Ambulates 8 feet and rests" says something definite and can be used as a point of comparison.

Once objective assessments have been charted, the next area to be covered is what the nurse is doing during the visit. This may involve a procedure or instruction or a combination of both. Again, the key is clarity. Muddy statements such as, "Instructed in effects and side effects of medication," or "Wound care done" are useless. These statements do not say anything. They are the home health equivalent of the night nurse in the hospital charting, "Quiet night, no complaints."

Specific instructions should be documented as they are taught. The nurse who instructs the patient in the side effect of medication should enter her specific instructions on the nursing note. Wound care should be documented with the same exact language. The use of sterile technique, the method of cleansing or debriding the wound, and the precise amount and type of dressing material used should be clearly noted on the visit note.

The next area on the visit note to be considered is the documentation of the patient's response. Again, vague, catch-all phrases should be avoided. Specific information is needed, such as, "Able to state times of medication administration and side effects of verapamil" or "Tolerates wound care without pain if acetaminophen taken one hour before care."

Home health nursing is an on-going process, and a plan for further care should be mentioned in every note. This may be very difficult if several nurses are seeing the patient, but it is not impossible. A plan does not have to be stated as an exact blueprint for the next visit. The plan can refer to areas of care or instruction that still need to be addressed. "Continue instruction in medications and begin diet instruction" can constitute a plan for further care. "Continue instructions to caregiver in wound care procedures" could be appropriate. The plan stated on the note should refer to specifics, taking into account the variables involved with both the patient and the nursing staff.

Writing a visit note does not have to be an ordeal if the nurse keeps a mental blueprint of method and content. The method described here starts with assessment and moves in sequence through actions taken, patient response, and plan. There are certainly other methods. The key is to find one and use it consistently. The content can be simplified if the nurse thinks in specific, objective terms and documents care in that manner, always keeping in mind that a good visit note must be able to be read, and not interpreted.

# Documentation in Home Care: Skilled Observation

*Elissa Della Monica, RN, MSN*
*Joan Yuan, RN, C, MSN*

Since the inception of the uniform physician plan of treatment forms (HCFA 485, 486, 487) for Medicare in September, 1985, home health agencies have been burdened with the cost of training staff to complete and process them. In addition, home health agencies have suffered a loss of or delay in reimbursement based on the fiscal intermediaries' review of these forms. Because nurses are expected to complete these forms according to Medicare specifications, it is of the utmost importance that they understand the relationship of the Medicare regulations to the accurate and timely completion of the physician's plan of treatment.

On form 486, nurses are asked to categorize clinical services within one of 27 designated treatment codes. These codes represent services to be rendered under the physician's plan of treatment (form 485). Agencies have been informed that the listing of a code for a particular service is not intended to imply coverage for these clinical services. According to the Medicare regulations,[1] a patient may qualify for skilled services if the following criteria are met: the patient must be homebound, care must be reasonable and necessary to the treatment of the patient's illness or injury, care is intermittent in nature, and the patient is under the care of a physician (signed plan of treatment certifies homebound status and need for skilled intermittent care).

In this column, we will discuss the application of the first treatment code (A-1), skilled observation. We will address the application and documentation of this treatment code within the framework of the nursing process: assessing, planning, implementing, and evaluating.

The Skilled Observation treatment code (A-1) is defined in the Medicare *Home Health Agency Manual* as: "All skilled observation of the patient where the physician determines that patient's condition is such that a reasonable probability exists that significant changes may occur which require the skills of a licensed nurse to supplement the physician's personal contacts with the patient."[1]

## ASSESSMENT

The assessment of the client by the nurse is the major component of the skilled observation treatment code. The assessment factors addressed during a skilled observation visit may include cardiovascular, respiratory, neurologic, genitourinary, gastrointestinal, musculoskeletal, and psychosocial components. For example, a patient with a diagnosis of acute congestive heart failure should have a thorough assessment of cardiovascular and respiratory systems, including vital signs, breath sounds, peripheral circulation, edema, and cyanosis. Medication regimen, signs and symptoms of complications, environmental safety and physical and psychologic restrictions of the disease process must also be included.

The nurse should be explicit in the documentation of the clinical assessment. The documentation should be structured in a manner that reflects how bad, not how good, the patient's status is. Medicare requires that the documentation reflect an instability in the disease process. In addition to that which is directly observed by the nurse, it is necessary to document the medical history relating to the instability of the disease state (eg, multiple cardiac arrests). This component is necessary because it enables the nurse to depict the patient's clinical status and, thereby, support the need for skilled services.

## PLAN

The plan must be specific to both the nursing and medical diagnoses. For example, a medical diagnosis of decubitus ulcer with a nursing diagnosis of actual impairment of skin integrity would have a plan that incorporates ongoing assessment of the decubiti, treatment of the decubiti, patient and family instruction, and ongoing evaluation of the treatment. The plan should explicitly describe care that requires the professional skills of a nurse because Medicare will make a determination of skilled services based on the complexity of the treatment plan and the description of the wound.

## IMPLEMENTATION

During the implementation phase, the nurse carries out the plan that he or she has established for the care of the patient. Throughout this phase, the nurse must be alert to changes in the patient's clinical status that would require a change in the treatment plan or require an alteration in the frequency and duration of the skilled nursing visits. This aspect of documentation is essential because the Medicare regulations state: "Where there has been no significant change (eg, no change in medication or vital sign stability, no recent exacerbation in the patient's condition) for a period of 3 weeks (or where the physician orders such services as infrequently as every 30 to 60 days) and no other necessary skilled nursing services are being furnished, nursing visits solely for observation and evaluation would not be considered reasonable and necessary."[1]

## EVALUATION

The evaluation of the effectiveness of the plan and its implementation is an ongoing process. The nurse must continually evaluate and document the patient's response. Is the unstable cardiac patient suffering side effects of a newly prescribed cardiac medication? Is the drainage from a wound becoming increasingly foul and copious? These types of changes would necessitate ongoing nursing and medical evaluation and communication with subsequent changes in the plan.

According to the Medicare regulations, a patient must be evaluated by a physician at least every 60 days.[1] When the physician sees the patient less frequently than once every 60 days, Medicare will question whether the patient is in need of the level of care that qualifies him or her for skilled nursing services.

If the nurse, through the mechanism of documentation, is able to demonstrate changes in the patient's clinical status with subsequent changes in the treatment plan, the care should be viewed as reasonable and necessary. This supposition, of course, is based on the patient meeting all other Medicare criteria for intermittent skilled care.

## CONCLUSION

The Medicare treatment code for skilled observation forms the basis for all skilled nursing care.  Because it may be the sole reason for the skilled visit or it may be provided in conjunction with other treatment codes, the documentation of skilled observation cannot be over-emphasized.  The nursing process of assessment, planning, implementation, and evaluation assists nurses in providing and documenting care in a manner that is consistent with Medicare regulations and professional nursing standards.

---

1. *Medicare Home Health Agency Manual.*  US Dept of Health, Education, and Welfare reprint 5.71.  Government Printing Office, 1966, pp 14.4-14.5.

# Documentation in Home Care: Teaching

*Marjorie McHann, RN, BS*

For teaching and training activities to be reimbursed, Medicare requires that the related coverage guidelines be fulfilled and be reflected in the nursing documentation. Therefore, it's important for you to be familiar with methods of documentation that reflect the guidelines, demonstrate the patient's need, and justify the teaching and training activities provided. How can your nursing documentation maximize reimbursement for teaching and training activities? Here are some tips.

*The patient's and/or caregiver's learning needs should be well documented.* The admission data base, the care plan, and the 486 clinical findings should identify learning needs that are pertinent to the patient's primary diagnosis and problems. Remember to relate the patient's knowledge deficit to a primary diagnosis and explain how it impedes recovery. You should leave no doubt about why teaching is needed and that it's likely to contribute to an improvement in the patient's condition or situation.

Take Mrs. Haversham's case . . . if her husband can learn how to do daily wound care on her infected leg ulcer, then it's likely that healing will be promoted. The 486 Update should say that: "Although Mr. Haversham was instructed in the hospital, he demonstrates inability to perform ulcer care satisfactorily in the home setting and needs further teaching. If husband can do daily leg ulcer care, healing will be promoted." This would help demonstrate that the teaching was reasonable and necessary and appropriate to Mrs. Haversham's illness.

*Document that the patient and/or caregiver is able, willing, and motivated to learn what you plan to teach.* Stipulate if there are any limitations that would affect the ability to learn, including physical, mental, or emotional disability. This information should be well documented in the admission data base, in the 486 Update and in subsequent summaries. By clearly and repeatedly documenting ability, willingness, and motivation to learn, you can demonstrate this coverage guideline is fulfilled and promote reimbursement for teaching visits.

*Your documentation should reflect the relationship between the diagnosis, the MD orders, the goals, the patient's condition, and teaching interventions.* Mr. Montazolli has acute congestive heart failure and cardiac arrhythmias and was admitted to the home health agency for skilled nursing visits. Let's see how the nursing documentation on Forms 485 and 6 helped maximize reimbursement for teaching visits.

- Form 485 listed his primary diagnoses as acute congestive heart failure and atrial fibrillation of recent onset.
- Form 485 MD Orders included teaching by the nurse that was consistent with his primary diagnoses. For example, orders were given for teaching related to the new cardiac medications: purpose, correct administration, and side effects.
- Form 485 Goals were also related to the primary diagnoses and doctor's orders. It was hoped, as a result of teaching, that Mr. Montazolli would be able to comply with his new medication regimen. This demonstrates how the teaching was expected to bring about an improvement in his condition.
- The admission clinical findings documented in the 486 Update also related to the primary diagnoses, doctor's orders, and goals. Thorough documentation of Mr. Montazolli's cardio-pulmonary status, problems, and related knowledge deficits helped to demonstrate that the teaching was reasonable and necessary.
- The 486 Update summary reflected that patient teaching was completed related to the purpose, correct administration, and side effects of Lanoxin, Lasix, and KCL.

By documenting that the teaching interventions were related to the diagnosis, orders, goals, and the patient's condition, it was demonstrated that the teaching visits were reasonable and necessary.

*Document all the teaching you do.* Be sure your teaching is clearly documented in the patient's visit note and in the 486 Update summaries. Remember, if it's not charted, it's not considered done!

Your documentation should specify exactly what teaching and training activities were provided. Be very specific about what was taught. You could chart, for example, that: "ADA diet teaching was continued related to food groups, allowed exchanges, and meal preparation."

To demonstrate that your teaching requires the specialized knowledge of a nurse, phrase your interventions in a way to emphasize the professional nature of the teaching. One way to accomplish this is to be very specific and use appropriate medical terminology.

Mrs. Haversham developed an upper respiratory infection. Her visit note might read: "Taught patient to force fluids." Or, it could say: "Taught patient need to increase PO fluids to 10 glasses a day to liquify bronchial secretions and facilitate expectoration." Without a doubt, the second note would fare much better in the hands of the reviewer!

*Demonstrate continuity of care in your documentation.* The visit notes, especially, should reflect an orderly flow to your teaching interventions. Don't jump around in your teaching. Your documentation should demonstrate that you followed the treatment plan. Anyone reading the patient's visit notes should be able to see that your teaching was logical, purposeful, and continuous.

Another important point about continuity... if teaching is interrupted for any length of time, be sure to give an explanation in your progress notes so it won't appear you just forgot.

Remember, by reflecting continuity in your documentation, you can help demonstrate that teaching was reasonable and necessary and promote reimbursement for teaching visits.

*Your documentation should also help maximize reimbursement for high frequencies.* If your patient has an acute learning need that requires intensive teaching visits 5, 6, or 7 times a week, then nursing documentation is even more important than ever. The clinical findings documented on the 486 Update must emphasize the patient's problems and give heavy justification for the need for frequent teaching visits. Leave no doubt why the teaching is needed and how it is expected to contribute to an improvement in the patient's condition.

Daily visits will be heavily scrutinized, and you should assume your visit notes will end up before the reviewer. More than ever, each visit note must stand on its own, demonstrating that the teaching done that visit was reasonable and necessary.

- Be sure each note reflects the patient's condition, the teaching, and the patient's response to the teaching.
- Document exactly what you teach each visit. Be very specific and use medical terminology that will emphasize the skilled nature of your teaching interventions.
- Document frequent contact with the physician in the visit notes.

By focusing on the patient's need, emphasizing the skilled nature of the teaching, and demonstrating continuing physician involvement, you can help demonstrate that daily teaching visits are reasonable and necessary.

*What about documentation of preventive teaching?* Preventive teaching is not covered by Medicare. To be reimbursed, teaching must be pertinent to the condition or diagnosis for which the patient is being seen. As you know, however, preventive teaching is essential to the overall well-being of the patient. It is a patient's right as well as the nurse's responsibility to teach precautions, preventive interventions, and wellness.

You can provide preventive teaching in conjunction with a nursing intervention that is considered skilled by Medicare. Include your preventive teaching on the visit note, but make certain the skilled service is well documented and evident to the medical reviewer. However, do not include the preventive teaching on Forms 485 and 6.

*Obtain MD orders for all your teaching.* The physician's orders on the 485 should reflect exactly what will be taught. It's not enough to say: "Teach ADA diet." Instead, say specifically what will be taught about the ADA diet, such as food groups, allowed exchanges, and meal preparation. This will promote reimbursement for teaching visits by emphasizing the skilled nature of the teaching and by helping to justify the frequency and duration of teaching visits.

In addition, if teaching by the nurse is required in response to patient problems that develop after admission, you must get a supplemental MD order. You'll recall that Mrs. Haversham developed an upper respiratory infection during her third week on service. For related teaching to be covered, it was necessary for the nurse to obtain a supplemental MD order documenting the new diagnosis of upper respiratory infection and specifically covering the related teaching activities.

Remember, for reimbursement, all care must be ordered by the physician.

*Document the patient's response to teaching.* As you know,

evaluation of the patient's response to teaching is an essential process. His nurse charted that: "Mr. Montazolli demonstrates good comprehension of teaching, as evidenced by his ability to recite the purpose and correct administration of Lasix." Also, in the visit notes and in the 486 Update summary, she reiterated the patient's response to teaching in terms of the goals that were set.

One of the Form 485 Goals was that, as a result of the teaching, Mr. Montazolli would be able to comply with the new medication regimen. She charted that: "As a result of teaching, Mr. Montazolli understands the purpose and correct administration of the Lasix and is now taking the medication as prescribed." By documenting Mr. Montazolli's response in this manner, she demonstrated the effectiveness of teaching interventions in terms of the goal that was set and justified the teaching activities provided.

Sometimes it's necessary to repeat or reinforce teaching due to a patient's slow learning abilities. In such cases, be sure to document in the progress note that the patient learns slowly; otherwise, visits to repeat or reinforce teaching may be denied. Medicare does not reimburse for repeated teaching or instruction unless you can document the necessity for continued teaching in the area.

Also, when documenting your teaching, the following words and phrases should be avoided: re-educated, reminded, reviewed, reinstructed, again instructed, urged, encouraged, and emphasized. These words serve as a red flag and might cause the reviewer to think that the teaching was repetitive, that the patient couldn't learn, or that the teaching was not reasonable and necessary.

In summary, for teaching and training activities to be reimbursed, your documentation must reflect the Medicare guidelines, demonstrate the patient's need for teaching, and justify the teaching and training activities provided. Remember, as long as your documentation supports the tests of reasonable and necessary, pertinence to the patient's condition, requiring the skills of a nurse, and ordered by the MD, teaching visits should be reimbursed.

In conclusion, home health nurses today must consider reimbursement when planning, implementing, and documenting teaching and training activities for home health patients. By practicing the principles of skilled documentation, you can reflect the Medicare guidelines, demonstrate the patient's need for teaching, and justify the teaching and training activities provided.

# Skilled Nursing HCFA-485 and HCFA-486 Tips

Patricia E. Harrison

Reprinted from *The Home Care and Documentation Guide*
by E.A. Huebner and P.E. Harrison, pp. 6:20-22,
with permission of Aspen Publishers, Inc., © 1991.

- Complete the patient's name and health insurance claim number (HICN) *exactly* as they appear on the patient's Medicare card. Verify for accuracy.

- If the patient is *over 100 years old*, mention this in the narrative statement in Item 22. The electronic screen may question the patient's eligibility (only the last two digits of the year are recorded), and this would satisfy the Medicare reviewer's question.

- Enter *all medications* and identify medications appropriately as new (N) or as changed (C). Remember to *update* on the recertification. If the patient has been on a medication for 60 days, it is no longer considered new. "New" orders involve medications that the patient has not taken recently (e.g., not within the last 30 days) or that the patient has never taken previously. "Change" orders involve changes in dosage, frequency, route, or time of administration within the last two months.

- The *principal diagnosis* is the diagnosis that accounts for the majority of home health services or visits. That diagnosis may not be the same as the principal diagnosis for the most recent hospitalization. For example, suppose a patient who was receiving PT services following a right below the knee (BK) amputation is hospitalized with pneumonia. The patient is discharged, requiring only two nursing visits for assessment of pulmonary status and medication teaching. However, the patient still requires extensive physical therapy services and an aide. The right BK amputation would remain the principal diagnosis and pneumonia would be added as a new secondary diagnosis.

• If possible, use diagnoses that are *acute* rather than chronic. It may be helpful to rephrase the diagnosis. Use onset dates within 60 days of admission to service, if possible. For example, instead of "COPD X 10 years," write "acute exacerbation of COPD 6/10/90." Exceptions to this include chronic conditions requiring ongoing skilled care, such as a catheter change for a neurogenic bladder, $B_{12}$ injections for pernicious anemia, or venipunctures for periodic bloodwork to monitor the patient's blood levels.

• *Qualify diagnoses* (e.g., unstable diabetes, uncontrolled hypertension). List as many diagnoses as apply that are related or contributory in order to support additional visits, if necessary.

• The *principal diagnosis* may change on a recertification if your primary reason for providing services to the patient changes due to an exacerbation of an existing condition or the development of a new problem. For example, suppose a patient with a right BK amputation is hospitalized for management of diabetes, and during hospitalization he becomes insulin dependent, requiring daily nursing visits upon discharge. Diabetes mellitus --insulin dependent would now be the new principal diagnosis.

Remember, if you change the principal diagnosis on a certification, be sure to change the ICD-9 code and date of onset accordingly.

• Another consideration in diagnosis selection is the use of *electronic screens* (the Wisconsin module) by fiscal intermediaries in reviewing claims. An electronic screen compares the diagnosis from the HCFA-485 against the accumulated numbers of visits by type and treatment codes from the HCFA-486. If the visits exceed the parameters for the diagnosis, the screen will reject the claim and a medical reviewer must then manually review the claim and approve or deny for payment. Selection of the appropriate principal diagnosis reflecting the most acute condition or the one for which the most services are being provided, can help your claim pass the electronic screen review. *The screens are only a guide.* They cannot be used to deny visits but only as an aid in claims processing. If a patient's condition warrants additional visits, they should be provided. Documentation must support the necessity of all visits.

• The following nine *V codes* are the most acceptable as principal diagnoses:

| V46.0 | Dependent on Aspirator |
| V46.1 | Dependence on Respirator |
| V53.5 | Fitting and Adjustment of Ileostomy or Other Intestinal Appliance |
| V53.6 | Fitting and Adjustment of Urinary Devices |
| V55.0 | Attention to Tracheostomy |
| V55.1 | Attention to Gastrotomy |
| V55.2 | Attention to Ileostomy |
| V55.3 | Attention to Colostomy |
| V55.4 | Attention to Other Artificial Opening of Urinary Tract |

All V codes are acceptable as secondary diagnoses and may assist in justifying the intensity of services being provided. For example, the administration of prednisone (V67.51) requires more intensive instruction and monitoring than most medications, and utilization of the V code as a secondary diagnosis makes it more likely a medical claims reviewer will notice prednisone is being used.

E codes are not acceptable as principal diagnoses.

• *Pay attention to the diagnosis.* If it is a diagnosis that does not usually render a patient homebound, explain why this particular patient is homebound. Coverage is unlikely if you simply list weakness, a speech problem, or senility. It is more effective to state, "Cannot ambulate without assistance of 1 person."

Remember, reviewers generally only have your written documents with which to judge the services you provide. Try to read your own notes objectively. do they really explain your patient's condition and justify the care you are providing? Is it clear why the spouse is not providing personal care and why the patient requires an aide?

• Enter the patient's *therapeutic diet* or the dietary requirements and restrictions and fluid needs as ordered by the physician. Remember that "no added salt," "low sodium," "no sugar," and "reduced fat" diets are not considered therapeutic diets. If necessary, inform the physician of this fact and seek clarification from the physician on specifically what type of diet and diet teaching the patient needs to achieve the desired goals. Only the teaching of specific therapeutic diets (e.g., "2-gm Na, 1500 calorie ADA") is covered as a skilled service under Medicare. The physician must order teaching services specifically (e.g., "Instruct patient on 1500 Cal ADA diet").

• List all *allergies,* including allergies to drugs, food, and environmental factors, such as dust and molds (HCFA-485, Item 17). They may justify increased teaching visits.

• *Functional limitations* and *activities permitted* assist in establishing homebound status and may justify a home health aide, teaching, and therapy services. It is important to show clearly all of the patient's functional limitations and to correlate them with the activities permitted. Be sure the activities permitted (HCFA-485, Item 18) do not contradict the functional limitations (Item 18A).

Do not feel restricted by the choices listed; utilize the "other" box, and add any additional information that will assist in demonstrating the patient's need for services, such as patient's inability to read. Provide a narrative explanation in Item 17 on the HCFA-486, if necessary.

• When describing the patient's *mental status,* consider the impact on the coverage of teaching services. If the patient is comatose or disoriented, a caregiver must be identified to justify the teaching. If the patient is disoriented and there is no caregiver, this would help to justify the services of a medical social worker. If the patient is forgetful, this would justify slower progress. If the patient is mentally limited or very anxious, this should be listed as "other" and a narrative explanation should be provided.

• If there is any *change in treatment* from the original plan of care (HCFA-485), be sure to obtain a signed physician's order (usually a short order form) and document the reason for the change on the HCFA-486 (Item 16). This would include any increase or decrease in visits or the addition of another discipline as well as any specific changes in the treatment plan.

• In filling in Item 22 of the HCFA-485 (Goals/Rehabilitation Potential/Discharge Plan), list *goals* that are realistic and pertinent to the diagnosis. Make sure the rehabilitation potential description is consistent with the prognosis. For example, if the prognosis is "poor," then how are you going to substantiate "significant improvement" in a reasonable amount of time? Would this be a realistic expectation? Don't forget to *describe* the rehabilitation potential. Just stating "fair" or "good" is inadequate. Be specific and exact, utilizing measurable terms and results that are attainable. *Example:* "Rehabilitation potential good to return to previous independence in self-care."

For discharge planning, reviewers want to see how the patient is expected to manage without home care. If you mention family members and the patient has an aide, is it clear why the aid is necessary? *Example:* "Patient to be discharged to self-care with assistance of spouse." From this example is it clear why the patient is currently receiving an aide?

• Catheter changes require a specific frequency, but a specific number of PRN visits can be added or a range of visits can be stated with PRN visits. *Example:* "1 x mo + 2 PRN for catheter problems" or "1-2 x mo + 2 PRN for catheter problems." Remember *PRN only orders do not meet the intermittent requirement.*

• For a catheter change, give the specific date and time of the change, the size of catheter, the number of cc's in the balloon, the appearance of urine, any problems, and any instructions provided. *Aides cannot change catheters.*

• Be absolutely positive that HCFA forms 485, 486, 487, and 488 (when requested) are consistent with the clinical and progress notes. Clinical notes must support all that is written on the HCFA forms. When form 488 is requested, it must be returned to the fiscal intermediary on a timely basis.

• In the case of vitamin $B_{12}$ injections, "1 x month" means just that -- it does not mean once every four weeks. Even with physician orders, any additional visits beyond the once-a-month maintenance dose for pernicious anemia would probably be denied. Remember, more frequent visits are acceptable in the initial stages of the diagnosis.

Evidence as to how the diagnosis was determined should be available in the agency chart (e.g., pernicious anemia -- Shilling test results). Upon the patient's admission to home care, request appropriate information from the hospital or physician to verify the diagnosis.

Remember, if the patient sees the physician once a month, the injection could be given by the physician and the home health visit may be denied.

• *Daily administration* of insulin is covered if the patient is incapable of self-administration and no one is available to perform this service. On each claim, document the patient's need for assistance in order to prevent questions from the medical claims reviewers. Documentation must reflect efforts to find someone capable of administering insulin to the patient.

Remember, there are syringes designed for visually impaired and blind diabetics. It is expected that these syringes will be obtained for a visually impaired diabetic. instructions for use would be considered a skilled service.

Prefilling syringes weekly is coverable in the following two circumstances:

1. A skilled service is required at least once every 60 days. It must be ordered and documented in addition to prefilling syringes. If a venipuncture for FBS is the *skilled* service, once every 60 to 90 days would suffice.
2. It is documented why patient is incapable of filling syringes and that there is no one else available to do it.

• *Medication charting* should include name, dosage, time of administration, route of administration, and site of injection. Chart responses or reactions to both the scheduled and unscheduled (PRN) medications. All drugs administered by the nurse, prescription as well as nonprescription medications, should be listed on the plan of care (HCFA-485) or be documented as specific verbal orders on the HCFA-486.

• The HCFA-485 should include any *dietitian services* ordered by the physician, even though they are not billable to the Medicare program, the costs are allowable and the provision of these services would need to be ordered by the physician. Some insurance companies pay for a dietitian's home visits.

• Information on the HCFA-485 series must be *consistent* with information submitted on the UB-82 (billing form) to ensure timely reimbursement. When discrepancies are identified, a HCFA-488 may be required.

• For patients receiving a high frequency of nursing and aide visits, the intermediary will count each visit as two hours to identify cases requiring medical review. Consequently, if the combined nursing and aide visits number more than 14, the claim will go to medical review. If the hours exceed 28 per week, they will be subject to closer scrutiny than if they are less than 28 per week. It is allowable to provide up to 35 hours of combined nursing and aide care and over 35 hours in "exceptional circumstances." The documentation on the HCFA-485 and HCFA-486 must justify that these services are reasonable and necessary.

# CHAPTER 3

# Clinical Management

# The Qualities of a Home Health Care Nurse

*Linda G. Cherryholmes*

Reprinted from Cherryholmes, L.G., The Qualities of a Home Health Care Nurse, *Home Health Care Nursing: Administrative and Clinical Perspectives,* S. Stuart-Siddall, ed. pp. 155-162, with permission of Aspen Publishers, Inc., © 1986.

This chapter addresses the unique qualities one would seek in a home health nurse. Numerous home health and hospital nurses were interviewed to see how they felt about this topic. Each was asked what "special qualities" were necessary to function well in her or his chosen role. Also queried were interviewers and supervisors, who usually conduct hiring interviews, as to what they look for in an interview that would make that person be a prime candidate for either a home health or a hospital nursing position. Clients were also queried about their view of the nurses who came to visit them.

Through the history and evolution of nursing there have been few changes in the basic principles and standards of nursing. Some of the most common and accepted standards are health promotion, health maintenance, health education, and disease prevention. Also acknowledged is the need for holistic and comprehensive planning for coordination and continuity of care. The nursing profession has gone through many changes in its process of evolution, and there has been a changing scope of nursing practice, with the trend toward increased specialization. Today's nurse can be a generalist or a specialist in the hospital as well as in the community health setting.

How does a nurse prepare for home health nursing? What does this specialty require? Is this a specialty within the framework of community health nursing, or a general area of its own with subspecialties? Does there need to be additional or specialized education? Does that body of knowledge have to come with the nurse, or can it be obtained as the nurse is oriented to home health? These are philosophical questions that are often asked. This chapter seeks to portray the uniqueness of the home health nurse.

Care in the community calls for a change in the basic attitudes on the part of many home health workers. There is a need to change the traditional modes of thinking in regard to the providers and recipients of care. Community health nursing services are directed toward developing and enhancing the health capabilities of people. The recipient of care, the client, has to be seen as part of the family and community. A holistic and humanistic philosophy of home care, the question of control and decision making, the family unity theme, and the crushing problem of paying for the many services are other areas that community nurses address.

## QUALITIES

The nurse in home health has to have a philosophy that is holistic, family-centered, broad, and nonjudgemental and must accept others and their value systems. The home care ethic contends that the client and the family unit come first. The nurse entering the home health field has to have the usual educational preparation, but experience in medical-surgical, rehabilitation, and gerontological nursing will greatly enhance the breadth of care delivered.

A humane approach is paramount in meeting the needs of ill people, especially in their home environment. Some factors that show that this nurse values providing quality care in a professional manner are the kind of life experiences she has had, her value system, and her awareness of self. Her knowledge also needs to encompass religious, ethnic, social, and economic influences that affect her client and family. Just within her visiting territory these can vary widely and be of such a diverse nature that her attention is required. The customs, mores, and traditions of the family have long been established and the nurse must be aware of this and proceed cautiously, rather than responding first to her own value system. Home health care is a total involvement with the client and family. They are to be dealt with on their own terms, in their own home, following their established habits and customs.

Out in the community, the nurse is alone on the client's turf. She cannot push, and has to know when to pull back. She has to like dealing with families. The whole family has to be involved in the care planning, along with the client, so that everyone shares the commitment of progress. The individual, the client, plays a central role, around which all else revolves. The home health nurse has to be able to be comfortable in nonstructured situations and to have an ability to relate to people in varied environments. The nurse has to be extremely tolerant of others' lifestyles and habits and to be aware that one cannot change the habits of a lifetime.

"Patience with our patients," is a saying to abide by, as well as, "love and respect the elderly." Respect their dignity, privacy, need for autonomy, and even the manner in which they are addressed. Such patients may tend to reminisce; one woman recited her medical history according to where she and her husband had been stationed during his 30-year military career — gallbladder trouble in Portsmouth, URIs in Boston, broken leg in San Francisco, and so on.

Other qualities are sensitivity, flexibility, adaptability, and a large dose of common sense. Empathy should be one of the strongest qualities of a home health nurse. Working one to one and understanding the client's problem and point of view are both elements of concern. It can be wearing on the nurse, and she has to give a great deal of herself in this role. The home health nurse works autonomously but at the same time has to be able to enlist the support, gain the cooperation, and have constant communication and rapport with the client, the family, and other health care professionals. There has to be confidence building to maximize the helping potential. She is in someone else's territory, and the main purpose is to assist the client and the family to function at their best possible level for preventing dependency. A fundamental of the nurse's practice would be health promotion activities that foster the client's well-being and that are aimed at preventing recurrence of illness.

The nurse has to feel comfortable with the unknown. One never knows what is behind that front door. A nurse is not a manager, nor is he or she in control of the situation or environment. The home health nurse has to be able to go into any type of environment or home and must be able to communicate on the appropriate level. There are many environmental distractions, and the nurse has to be able to work with and withstand the elements of nature and various creatures of nature. There is an awareness of the total environment and its influences. Also, she has to be adaptable to the environment. She can go from a less than desirable neighborhood to one of the finest. She needs to be streetwise, to know the safest way to walk and drive within her area and how to handle herself in different neighborhoods. She must have a knowledge of ethnic cultures, ways, and mores, know that certain behaviors and actions that are acceptable with one culture are unacceptable with another. It is beneficial if a nurse can speak another language, especially in communities that have large populations of foreign-speaking people.

The home health nurse has to be able to accept the clients' perceptions and the reality of their environment and lifestyle. A knowledge of the overall needs of the person is very important. In the home situation, the nurse is more intimately involved. She learns the inner workings of the family because she is in close contact over a longer time span than in a hospital. It is a more relaxed environment, and a personal relationship develops with the client and the family. She deals much more with the emotions of everyday.

The nurse must be able to terminate the therapeutic relationship effectively. This can be difficult owing to the investment of energies on the part of both the nurse and the client. It can be likened to seeing one's firstborn go to the first day of school. The goal has been the client's independence, to function the best he or she can with what he or she has, but it is also a trifle sad because so much love, caring, concern, and commitment have been expended to reach this point.

## ABILITIES OR STRENGTHS

More technical skills are needed today. The home health nurse is a higher-leveled generalist who has to be able to recognize problems and trust her own judgement and clinical skills. Knowledge of norms is necessary because there is no peer just down the hall with whom to corroborate.

Fine assessment skills are crucial. The nurse has to be able to assess the client's response to medications, treatment, teaching, and changes in physical status. The nurse is a teacher and has to have the ability to think on her feet as to when the prime and optimum moment for teaching is most beneficial. There can be flexibility in this because of the visit schedule. A small amount of teaching can be done at each visit, and the nurse will be able to see how much the client is learning. She can look for feedback and give reinforcement when progress has been made. The home health nurse has to plan ahead, to determine what the goals are, what will be covered this visit and the next. Then, how is she going to assist the client to achieve his or her goals? She must be independent in her nursing functions, have keen and reliable judgement, with faith in her own abilities.

She is a problem solver and seeks, first, to assist the client in identifying the problem and then work through the problem-solving process. She should be familiar with the concept of change. Being able to use the dynamic forces that influence change is a vital part of the totality of working in community health. She has to be able to assist the client to see the need for change and then help the client through the change process.

She has initiative and is a self-starter. There has to be some flexibility in being able to deal with and treat people with challenging cases and situations. The nurse needs to have the ability to organize. Often she sets up her own schedule regarding visits, the number of visits per week, and the number of clients seen per week and per day. Also necessary is the ability to schedule for the convenience of the client as well as for the individual nurse. Truly necessary in home health is the ability to read a map, to have a sense of direction, and to be able to navigate. There are many other qualities for a home health nurse, such as versatility and systems savvy, which is a knowledge of the health care bureaucracy and how to work with it and within it. The home health nurse also needs to have the ability to make decisions, to be cost-conscious, innovative, and able to improvise.

## LIMITATIONS

There is less one-on-one supervision in home health. The team leader or head nurse is not just down the hall. Also, there is far less peer support. The nurse cannot go around the corner to a peer to ask a question. True, there is a supervisor available by phone, if the client happens to have a telephone. Resources are not as readily available. There is no med room, nor is there a central supply in another part of the building. Medical libraries, journals, peers, or consultants are not in the same area with the home health nurse. There is no one at that time with whom to discuss thoughts or ideas. Also the nurse does not have backup physically present. It is in the office, but it is not nearby and there is no "next shift" to carry on. She has to do her work and do it in a complete manner and then move on to the next client, but each of her clients is her responsibility. Some environmental distractions can be extremely uncomfortable, such as safety, weather, neighborhoods, and creatures. If she cannot accept the habits of others, then home health may not be the field for her. Homes can be dirty and have a number of nature's creatures roaming about freely. Another limitation is that one does establish a close and oftentimes long-term relationship with the client and family, and sometimes that empathy can lead to sympathy, which can then be an interference.

## ROLES

The nurse in home health plays multiple roles. This person wears many hats. She is part social worker, financial counselor, dietitian, consumer/client advocate, teacher, case manager, and coordinator. Many of the rose overlap. The home health nurse has to be self-reliant and have the ability to pace. It is imperative that she remain the client advocate and realize that her role is as coordinator, that she does not overstep her bounds. At times there is a fine line between nursing and medical judgement. She is a friend, a spiritual comforter, a psychologist to the client and family. She is also a physical therapist, an occupational therapist, and a translator of medical information. Another role is that of facilitator, because the client is the one with the active role, and the home care nurse seeks to assist the client to achieve the goal of positive health behaviors. It is necessary to nurture and develop an interrelationship.

There are many aspects of direct care, such as assessment, treatments, teaching, a role model for positive health behaviors, and technical skill. The home health nurse needs to have a knowledge base of the regulatory mechanisms and the methods of reimbursement that determine what is a skilled service so that the agency can receive reimbursement. There are many aspects of indirect care — consultation with other health personnel, staffings, team conferences — as everyone works together to facilitate the client in achieving the highest level of wellness.

## INTERACTIONS

Communication skills are prime in the role of the home health nurse. She and the other team members convey an attitude of warmth, caring, and kindness. One of the goals is to assist the client to understand the "why" of the treatments and what is necessary to achieve wellness.

The home health nurse is a relatively independent practitioner. There is a multidisciplinary team, true, but it is not a team as in a hospital The physician remains the "coach" of the team, but the nurse is the quarterback who coordinates and uses the strengths of the other team members.

Caution is essential to avoid using the label of "noncompliance." Give the client the benefit of the doubt. He may desire to comply, but some factor is influencing his ability not to comply. Seek to unearth the elusive factor. Because someone chooses against what we believe to be right doesn't mean they are noncompliant. Remember, you are their advocate; I may not agree with you, but I'll support your right of choice.

In working with the client and family, teaching them, and gaining their cooperation, the home health nurse has to be able to assimilate data and then communicate it concisely to the physician and other members of the health care team. The nurse must be able to develop a working relationship with others to promote coordinated and thoughtful action.

The goals must be mutually established; they should not be just the nurse's goals but should be based on the client's perception of the situation. The nurse and client should agree mutually; then, it is hoped, there will be better compliance owing to an ownership of the goals; the client will then strive to meet them with greater enthusiasm. The nurse has to be accepting of the client's right to self-determination regarding decision making, and his decision may be not to comply with the treatment. A question that may be asked is, "How much noncompliance can the team tolerate?"

## NURSING PLAN

The home health nurse has a broad knowledge of community resources. She is a practiced and skilled diplomat, is able to assess and weigh alternatives and choose the best course of action for all concerned while maintaining objectivity. The nurse has the ability to assume the role of others temporarily with direction from the supervisor or administrator, especially if nursing responsibilities are unclear or seem inappropriate. The concept of case management establishes a system of appraisal, care planning, and care evaluation. There is an enhancement of the continuity of care, and all care providers should describe the client in identical terms. In the case management system there is a professional plan to meet the individual's needs. A written plan of action is imperative to ensure that tasks are carried out, that established standards are complied with, and that there is a continuous reassessment and evaluation.

The nursing process is ever ongoing, with constant reassessment, reordering of priorities, and then new mutual goal setting and revision of plan. It is imperative to tailor the nursing plan to the client and the client's environment. Using the nursing process is a way to ensure the current client need while anticipating needs that may surface in the future. Case management is a coordination of the work of various disciplines in reducing health risk, and it is usually the nurse who coordinates because she is usually the person who opens the record. The nursing process is extremely valuable, especially the reassessment and reevaluation phases to modify plans as needed.

## CONSUMER

New habits of self-reliance and self-care have to be learned, and the client has to incorporate wellness, preventive health, and holistic care in his or her daily life. The nurse is a role model for these positive health behaviors. The consumer is provided with data needed to make informed decisions about promoting, maintaining, and restoring health, about seeking and using appropriate health care resources.

## SYSTEMS

Utilization of a systems approach is one of the primary foundations of community health. There are social systems and subsystems; all have a mutual respect for the rights and obligations of others. There are many players in this system and, one hopes, a willingness to address the major issues. There are many alliances and supportive networks to be developed. An objective of the home health nurse is to determine the power structure of all the systems — the agency, the client, the family, and the other members of the health care community. The interactions of the team are prime in order to render the finest care in an efficient and cost-effective manner.

## SUMMARY

The home health nurse is a caring, autonomous, and

accountable professional. This nurse values the client and the behaviors that promote the highest level of wellness for the individual. The focus of care is on disease prevention and health maintenance. The dynamics of interactions are paramount — among the client, the family, and the multidisciplinary health care team. As with nurses in other specialty areas, certain qualities are unique to the home health nurse.

---

**BIBLIOGRAPHY**

American Nurses' Association. *Standards of Community Health Nursing Practice.* Kansas City, Mo.: ANA, 1973.
——. *A Conceptual Model of Community Health Nursing.* Kansas City, Mo.: ANA, 1980.
——. *A Guide for Community-based Nursing Services.* A draft document. Kansas City, Mo.: ANA, 1984.
Arbeiter, Jean S. "The Big Shift to Home Health Nursing." *RN* 47 (1984): 38-45.
Cobb-McMahon, Barbara A., David D. Williams, and Joy Hastings Davis. "Changing Health Behavior of Community Health Clients." *Journal of Community Health Nursing* 1 (1984): 27-31.
De Crosta, Tony, ed. "Home Health Care: It's Red Hot and Right Now." *NursingLife* 4 (1984): 54-60.
Florida Nurses Association. *Position Statement on the Role of the Community Health Nurse.* Orlando, Fla.: Florida Nurses Association, 1984.
Grau, Lois. "What Older Adults Expect from the Nurse." *Geriatric Nursing* 5 (1984): 14-18.
Mayers, Marlene. "Home Visit-Ritual or Therapy?" *Nursing Outlook* 21 (1973): 328-331.
Spiegel, Allen D. *Home Healthcare.* Owings Mills, Md.: National Health Publishing, 1983.
Stanhope, Marcia, and Jeanette Lancaster. *Community Health Nursing: Process and Practice for Promoting Health.* St. Louis: C.V. Mosby Co., 1984.
Stewart, Jane Emmert. *Home Health Care.* St. Louis: C.V. Mosby Co., 1979.
Weinstein, Sharon M. "Specialty Teams in Home Care." *Nursing84* (1984): 342-345.

# Home Visiting Steps

*Carolyn J. Humphrey*
*Paula Milone-Nuzzo*

Used with Permission, Humphrey, C. and Milone-Nuzzo, P.,
*Home Care Nursing: An Orientation to Practice.*
Norwalk, CT: Appleton & Lange, 1991.

Steps of the home visit are broken down into three stages, each with activities that must be accomplished before another stage is begun. The three stages are:

1) the pre-visit stage
2) the visit stage
3) the post-visit stage

Each stage will be described and discussed in this section. The stages of the home visit, with specific activities are summarized in Figure 2-4.

**The Pre-Visit Stage.** The pre-visit stage includes activities that prepare the home care nurse to accomplish the tasks of the home visit. The first step of this stage is to familiarize yourself with the client's chart and the purpose of your home visit. This is helpful in planning your day since some clients will require visits at specific times, and some visits will take longer than others. For example, if the chart indicates that the purpose of the home visit is to observe the client administer her morning insulin, clearly the home care nurse needs to be at the client's home early in the morning. In some cases, clients have sophisticated and complex procedures that need to be done. By reviewing the chart, the home care nurse can plan to spend the needed time with the client.

An important pre-visit activity is the telephone call to the client to confirm the visit. In most cases of follow-up visits, the home care nurse has planned with the client at the previous visit when subsequent visits will be made. Even though this may have been done previously, it is essential that the client be called to confirm that he is expecting a visit and that the time of the visit is convenient. This telephone call should be brief, but it is useful to ask the client how he or she is feeling and if there has been a significant change in the client's condition since the last home visit. Avoid allowing the client to go into a long description of all his or her health problems, and tell him or her that you will be there shortly to discuss it. If there has been a change in the client's condition, you can plan for this visit more easily before leaving the office. Perhaps you will need to review some books to determine the proper assessment or intervention, or perhaps a case conference with your supervisor is indicated.

Once the home visit is planned and confirmed by the telephone call, a thorough review of the chart takes place. You need to be thoroughly familiar with the client's history, medical problems, medication regime, and care plan with special attention given to the client's specific interventions. Your supervisor or another nurse may be instrumental in filling you in on some aspects of the

---

**Figure 2-4. The Home Visiting Process**

Pre-visit activities
Familiarize yourself with the client's chart
Telephone call to the client to confirm visit and time
Thorough review of the client's chart
Arrange necessary equipment for the visit
Review the route to the client's home
Leave schedule for the day at the agency

Visit Activities
Social phase (brief)
Wash hands and arrange equipment
Implement activities of care plan
Gather equipment and wash hands
Plan for next home visit

Post-visit activities
Revise care plan, if needed
Documentation
Communication with members of the health care team
Referrals, if indicated
Care for used equipment
Replenish nursing bag

case, but a thorough review of the chart should provide you with the information you need. (This makes a strong case for good documentation!) From this review, you can plan the agenda of your visit. If you are unfamiliar with a medication or specific intervention, go to a nursing text. Before entering the client's home you should have a mental picture of how the visit will unfold, but always remain flexible since priorities and clients' needs change and this affects the course of the home visit.

The next pre-visit activity is checking your nursing bag and arranging the necessary equipment. If your agency uses nursing bags, it is your responsibility for keeping the bag well stocked and in good condition. There are certain items basic to all nursing bags, and they are listed in Figure 2-5. Since you have reviewed the interventions that need to be accomplished, additional necessary equipment can be easily assembled. For example, if you know that a blood sugar is needed for Mr. Brown as part of his care plan, you must plan do a blood test on this visit and take a glucometer with you.

---

**Figure 2-5. The Contents of the Nursing Bag\***

Soap
Paper Towels
Forceps
Scissors
Thermometers (oral and rectal)
Cotton balls
Tongue depressors
4 x 4 gauze
Gauze
Gloves - clean (ample supply)
Sterile gloves (one pair)
Apron
Syringe-needles (assorted lengths and gauges)
Tape
Alcohol wipes
Tape measure
Flashlight
Stethoscope and sphygmomanometer
Map
Copy of Home Care Nursing

---

\* This is a list of the standard equipment that is part of all home care nursing bags. Your agency may have additional items that nurses are required to carry and that may need special standing orders (e.g., adrenaline).

Before you leave the agency, the route to the client's home should be reviewed. You should always carry a map, but if the map is reviewed in the agency and directions are written out, the chances of getting lost are reduced. It is important that directions to the client's home be written on the record of admission. If this is done consistently, subsequent visits are easier and quicker.

You will need to leave your proposed daily schedule at the agency so you may be reached while you're out. Some agencies use a tickler system that consists of a small box and 3 X 5 cards, each with the name of a client on it. The tickler box is divided with index cards for each day of the month. As the nurse sees a client, the index card is filed behind the index card for the date of the next scheduled home visit. In this way, clients don't get lost and the scheduled visits for a specific day are easy to identify. Other agencies ask the nurses to fill out a route slip with the client's name and anticipated visit time. Many agencies use computers to assist with this function. This activity is more important than it may seem. Sometimes a client will call the agency to cancel a visit or a physician will call with new orders after a nurse has left for the day. By knowing where the nurse is, the supervisor can call the preceding patient and leave that message. On a more personal note, you may need to be reached while in the field for a personal emergency, so if care is taken with your schedule the supervisor will have little difficulty reaching you.

**The Visit Stage.** The initial face-to-face meeting between the nurse and the client is very important since it sets the tone for the relationship to follow. The first few minutes of the home visit are generally viewed as the social phase, when the client and the home care nurse may have some light conversation so that both are put at ease. After this phase, the nurse is ready to begin to implement the care plan. As discussed before, the equipment you need on the home visit will usually be carried in your nursing bag. Although "bag technique" is often thought of as an old fashioned concept, it is an important part of asepsis in the home. Techniques for the use and care of the nursing bag are essential to reduce the spread of organisms from one client to another, from nurse to client, or from client to nurse. The following steps in bag technique should be used on every visit to maximize the efficient and effective use of the nursing bag.

*Bag Technique*

1. Place the bag in a clean area, preferably on a wooden table. If a clean area cannot be found, the bag should always be placed on something like a newspaper to avoid contaminating the outside of the bag. Do not place your bag on stuffed furniture or at a level where an inquisitive child or pet can gain access to the bag and contaminate it or harm themselves. Always keep your bag in sight.
2. Select something that will be used to discard contaminated equipment, such as a paper or plastic bag, or a bag made from newspaper.
3. Wash your hands using the soap and paper towels in your bag. It is always best to use your own soap and towels unless the patient has paper towels for your use. Do not use a cloth towel unless the patient has one for your use only. Leave the equipment at the sink until the end of the visit.
4. Only now, after handwashing, can the nurse enter the bag and take out the equipment needed for the visit. Place the equipment on a clean paper towel.
5. Proceed with the visit and discard dirty equipment into the paper or plastic bag. If syringes are used, you should know the agency's procedure for discarding them. Check this procedure with your supervisor before making home visits. If there is an unusually large, contaminated dressing, another bag may be needed. The family should be taught how to discard all dirty equipment safely.
6. When the visit is completed, clean the used equipment and wash your hands before replacing equipment in the bag. Never reenter the bag unless you have washed your hands.
7. Close the bag and leave it in a clean area until you are ready to leave.

**REMEMBER**

- The contents of the bag are considered clean. When items from the bag are used, they must be cleaned before they are put back in the bag (see section on universal blood and body fluid precautions.)
- The floor is considered a dirty area — never put you bag on the floor.
- Newspaper is considered clean and can be used if other items, such as bags, are unavailable.

- Place handwashing supplies — soap and paper towels — at the top of the bag where they can be easily reached.
- When not in use, the bag should be kept latched. Keep the bag out of sight when traveling in the car. Bring the bag in at the end of the day since extremes in temperature can damage equipment.
- Avoid bringing the bag into particularly dirty homes or where a client has a communicable disease. Prepare a small bag with the specific equipment you will need. Include in that bag, another bag in which to put back your cleaned equipment.
- Use the client's equipment as much as possible.

As mentioned, you will begin the intervention part of the visit by using the soap in the nursing bag and washing your hands. Always wash your hands before starting the visit. Following the handwashing procedure, the implementation of the care plan begins with such activities as teaching, direct care (e.g., a wound dressing), or assessment of the client's physiological or psychosocial status. While coordinating these activities, the home care nurse is constantly observing the client, the family, and the environment to determine if some modifications need to be made in the plan of care. It is important that the home care nurse involve the client and family or the significant other at every step of the implementation process. If the primary purpose of the visit is for the home care nurse to perform a dressing change, the nurse can be describing the procedure or the wound as the care is being performed. This will help the client and family to feel like active participants in the care. Once the implementation of the care plan is complete, the nurse should gather any equipment used and wash her hands. If equipment, such as thermometers, need to be washed or disposed of, it can be done at this time also.

In closing the visit, you will want to review the care the client is assuming or any aspects of the care plan that are particularly confusing. You will also set up an appointment for the next home visit and remind the client that he will receive a telephone call on the day of the visit to confirm the appointment. Although clients may devise their own system of remembering when visits are scheduled, if a client is having a particularly difficult time remembering when the home care nurse will come, marking a large calendar with the visit days is often useful.

**The Post-Visit Stage.** The home visit is not complete at the time you leave the client's home. Many activities comprise the post-visit stage and need to be done before your responsibilities are fulfilled. Based on the data collected during the home visit, revisions of the care plan may be indicated. You may have identified a new problem that should be added to the problem list and documented in the record, or resolved a problem that should be noted as such. Revision of any and all aspects of the care plan is completed following the home visit.

One of the most significant activities in the post-visit stage is the documentation of the interaction. Not only does documentation allow for communication between nurses and other health care providers, it provides the basis for reimbursement. There are many ways that documentation is accomplished, and you need to be thoroughly familiar with the system used by your agency.

An important post-visit activity is the communication of important information to other health care providers working with the client. It is during this stage that you may need to call the primary care provider to report the client's current condition. Case conferences with other disciplines involved (e.g., physical therapy, occupational therapy, social worker, nutritionist) may occur during this stage. Intra-agency communication is also a necessary part of this stage. If another nurse is serving as primary care nurse for the client, a brief verbal report of the visit is indicated, but the documentation on the client's chart should outline what was done on the visit and the client's status. At times, a report to the nursing supervisor is also indicated.

Referral to community agencies is also a part of post-visit activities. For example, if you determine that a client needed Meals on Wheels, you may make the referral in the client's home or wait until returning to the agency. Remember, always ask permission to use the client's telephone and make only local calls. If there is a chance that the referral source will ask for information that should not be stated in front of the client or family, make the referral at the agency.

Finally, you must care for any equipment that is to be returned to the agency and replenish your nursing bag with equipment and supplies. An ample supply of soap, paper towels, aprons, and other disposable supplies should be in your bag at all times. Agency policy will identify specific items to be carried in your bag. It is most helpful to replenish the bag at the completion of the home visit rather than at the beginning of the next day since you will have a clear memory of what equipment was used that day.

The home visit is the single most important tool for a home care nurse. As a guest in the client's home, you must recognize how certain behaviors have an impact on the implementation of the client's care. There are three phases in the home visit process; pre-visit activities, visit activities, and post-visit activities. The effective use of the nursing bag involves a technique that is carried out in a logical way during every visit. If all the phases of the home visit process are carried out in order, you will become an efficient and effective practitioner of home care nursing.

# Priorities

*Pat Carr, RN*

More and more frequently, the field nurse admitting a patient to the services of a home health agency may feel as if he or she is walking into a minefield. The population is aging and medical technology is continually improving. As a result, more and more patients are at home, managing multiple medical problems with the assistance of family members. When the home health agency is involved, the nurse must be able to quickly and accurately determine how to set priorities for the care and teaching to be done.

When setting priorities, the nurse must take into account the abilities of the patient and caretaker, the patient's diagnosis, the family support system, the available community resources, and the assistance that can be provided by the agency. All of this must be done quickly to ensure the patient's safety at home and to provide a blueprint for the care to be given.

One system of setting priorities involves placing the patient and family needs into five categories. This system allows for both agency and community assistance and is flexible enough to respond to changing patient needs. The five categories include immediate goals to be addressed on the first visit, short-term goals that can be met with agency assistance, short-term goals to be met by the patient or family, long-term goals that can be met with agency assistance, and long-term goals to be met by the patient and family.

What does this patient have to know before my next visit? The answer to this question will help the nurse to determine the immediate needs of the patient. Emergency phone numbers must be posted. The patient or a family member must be aware of any life-threatening complications that could occur, and must know what actions to take in that event. The patient who is at risk for an episode of acute pulmonary edema must know the signs and must know what actions to take. Safety must be addressed. There must be a means of communication with the health care team. The patient must be able to safely transfer to a bedside commode. Procedures must be considered. For example, the patient with a Foley catheter must be able to empty the drainage bag. The patient who is home with a new colostomy must be able to drain or empty the appliance pouch. Since the patient or caregiver will have to give medications, a schedule must be set up. Depending on the frequency of nursing visits, the nurse can make judgements as to what has to be dealt with. The first visit should not be concluded until the patient or family is able to deal with acute problems that might arise at any time.

Before the second visit, the nurse can evaluate and prioritize patient needs into the four remaining categories. Needs that can be addressed as short-term goals with agency assistance include anything that the nurse perceives will become a patient or family responsibility within one to three weeks. Wound care may be initiated by the nurse and taught to the family. Personal care can be managed with the assistance of a home health aide until the patient is able to participate. Instructions in procedures and disease process may be taught to the family or patient with the nurse continuing to evaluate the patient's clinical status.

Independent short-term goals include those daily tasks that will quickly become the responsibility of the patient and family. Safe transfers for toileting, daily skin care and observation for pressure ulcers, and daily weights fit into this category. These needs must be addressed during the first week of service. Technique and understanding can be assessed by the nurse during the skilled visit, but the actual activity must be done by the patient or family.

Eventually, responsibility for all care must be assumed by the patient and family. Long-term goals can also be split into those achievable with agency assistance and those that must be met independently. Long-term goals that are achieved with agency assistance involve referrals. If assistance with personal care will be an ongoing need, referral to community resources or private agencies may be necessary. A diabetic patient may benefit from further instruction in managing the disease once he or she is no longer homebound. A referral to an outpatient group might be helpful. These goals can be met with agency assistance, frequently by involving a social worker in the patient's care.

Long-term goals to be realized independently by the patient and caregiver include a thorough knowledge of disease management, medication administration, and side effects, therapeutic diet planning, and any ongoing procedures. While nurses address these points throughout their visits with patients, they may choose to concentrate more heavily on them after all of the short-term goals are met.

The setting of appropriate goals and priorities of care is essential in home health nursing. Except during brief nursing visits, the patient and family are essentially "on their own" and must be given the knowledge and skills to provide safe and appropriate care. For the patient with multiple medical problems, priority setting is particularly important. The use of the five categories described can provide an organized simple approach that recognizes all of the patient needs and deals with them according to urgency. In other words, the use of the five categories can provide a map to guide patient and nurse safely through the minefield of complex care.

# Productivity

*Carolyn J. Humphrey*
*Paula Milone-Nuzzo*

Used with permission, Humphrey, C. and Milone-Nuzzo, P.,
*Home Care Nursing: An Orientation to Practice.*
Norwalk, CT: Appleton & Lange, 1991.

Increasing concern about health care costs and the need to control factors that improve efficiency have increased the focus on productivity in home health agencies. The discussion of productivity and visit standards need not conjure up negative responses from staff members within an agency if everyone understands the reasons why productivity and visit standards are so important to a home health agency. First, no agency can survive without at least breaking even on expenses and income, and to do that, personnel must be efficient. Second, the agency wants to assure quality, and monitoring productivity can increase the likelihood that staff members are providing high-quality care.

Although productivity is difficult to measure in health care, it is not impossible, and many home health agencies have developed ways to reach this goal. Before the home care nurse can become familiar with the productivity standards used in an agency and understand how they are applied, she must understand the following productivity concepts summarized here from Benefield's (1988) work:

- Productivity is the relationship between the use of resources and the results of that use.
- Efficiency is not necessarily how fast work is done, but how well time is used.
- Quality can improve at the same time that productivity increases.

- Improving productivity involves all departments in a home health agency, never just one department or staff.
- Productivity is a "people issue," and since approximately 80% of a home health agency's budget is spent on personnel, *all* agency personnel contribute to productivity.
- Hands on skills are very important, but so also is the home care nurse's ability to think critically, solve problems, and make decisions that impact on the total care the client receives. These attributes must be factored into productivity issues.
- Visit standards should be developed that consider the intensity of service provided to the client (complexity level of the client), and the case mix (types of clients) of the population served by the agency. They should also take into consideration the efficiency of the paper flow in the total organization.
- Effectiveness of the service is an important productivity component and a crucial aspect of the agency's quality assurance program. The expectations of the outcomes of the home visit as well as the standards set for what is to go on in a home visit are important parts of understanding productivity in home care.

## FACTORS THAT AFFECT PRODUCTIVITY

A staff nurse should be constantly looking for ways to work smarter, not harder. Studies of the professional productivity conclude that the focus should not be on working faster (rushing through visits) but on using time efficiently and spending time doing those skills that the nurse was trained to do (Benefield, 1988). This is an important concept for all employees of the agency to remember, and it can be helpful when finding ways to help others be more efficient. There are several factors that can that can be considered to increase productivity.

**Case Load Management.** The case load is a group of clients assigned. For a primary nurse, a case manager, or a team leader, the case load will be the clients whose care she must direct. As a member of the team, the case load will be the case(s) assigned for a given time period, such as a day, week, or whatever the length of time the client is on service. The way that the work relating to these clients is organized is termed case load management.

There are many factors that affect the nurse's ability to manage a case load including:

1. The frequency (number of times a week) and length (visit time) of visits to the case load clients
2. The specific needs of the clients in the case load (i.e., teaching, direct care, coordinating multi-agency involvement, and psychosocial involvement). This can be visit- or nonvisit-related time.
3. The level of difficulty of the clients in your case load. This is usually determined by a client classification system used in the agency that categorizes the level of acuity experienced by clients using several different variables.

Each agency should have systems in place to help the nurse learn skills of case load management. The best resources for learning case load management are scheduling conferences with a supervisor about client issues and working with experienced nurses who can share the ways they have found to be more efficient. Also, by using the strategies outlined in the home visiting section of Chapter 2, and the suggestions listed in the following pages about contracting and patient teaching, the nurse will be able to develop her case load management skills.

**Work Load Management.** Work load is a summary of all the activities of a home care nurse, including case load management. Each agency should have a process for analyzing a nurse's work load often through the use of forms to be completed or interactions with the nursing supervisor. In addition to the material collected for measuring the case load management activities, the nurse will be recording the time spent on activities other than home visiting. These can include agency activities such as in-service programs, staff meetings, and conferences; community activities such as clinics or committee work; work in off-site areas such as schools; and personal time such as lunch, holidays, and vacations.

The new staff nurse may not be familiar with keeping track of her daily time in this manner. She would be assured that she is asked to do this, not because of agency distrust, but because the nature of home care is independent, and the agency needs to collect this information to justify costs to regulatory bodies and for budgeting purposes. Federal agencies, such as the Internal Revenue Service and the Social Security Administration, also require that this information be recorded. It is important that this information be accurate and up-to-date to be fair to the nurse and to the agency.

**Time Management.** The only manager of a home care nurse's time is the nurse. To be effective and efficient in professional practice, the nurse must be insightful concerning her use of time. The new home care nurse will identify many items that are time-wasters or time-savers, adding to the list that may have been started earlier in her career. Home care is a very independent practice, and the nurse must use self-discipline and motivation to stay efficient. The use of contracting, outlined in this chapter, is the best time-saver a home nurse can use in clinical practice working directly with clients. There are other ways to manage time effectively and they are listed below.

- Schedule clients who live in close proximity to each other together to minimize travel time.
- Keep a daily file to identify clients that need to be seen and other activities planned for certain days. A tickler card file or a calendar appointment book can be used to keep information from becoming misplaced. This is important so that planned visits are kept track of, and clients are seen on time.
- Find a quiet place to do your recording. This is not always easy in a small office that has a lot of distracting activity going on. If possible, documentation should be completed in the client's home during the visit or immediately after the visit. Many nurses find restaurants in their visiting area that offer enough space and privacy to do their paperwork while the nurse has a soft drink or cup of coffee. If most of the nurse's visit recording is completed before her return to the office, she will be better prepared for the other work activities that await her and the quality of the recording will improve because the information will have been recorded when it was clear in her memory.
- Charting should be done so well that few additional notes are needed. The recording should be complete enough that if there must be communication with others, such as social workers or physical therapists, the client's record should include the bulk of the required information. Nurses are notorious for repeating orally what they have written (or should have written) in the record — a carry over from the change-of-shift-report. This is a waste of time, especially in home care.
- Limit socializing. Most of the workday is spent with clients not colleagues, so it is important to make time to socialize with coworkers. The nurse must determine when that will be and for how long. Meeting with other nurses for lunch can often be

a positive use of time while it frees up the time in the office for work-related issues.

- Keep phone time to a minimum. Make all telephone calls in one block of time as much as possible, and always have something to work on (e.g., a client record) while on hold. Prepare an agenda for phone conversations to avoid forgetting any pieces of information.

- Delegate work to others. The agency employs support staff that are available to free the nurse up for nursing-related functions. The staff nurse should look for ways to improve the quality of interaction among agency staff members, through constructive feedback to the supervisor and in staff meetings. Remember, when a nurse identifies a problem area it is up to her also to develop ways to solve it and then become committed to making the approach work.

- Always call clients and give them an approximate time for the home visit (e.g., late morning, early afternoon). Do not predict a precise arrival time since scheduling is based on estimated time spent on earlier visits, and the nurse does not want to set up a situation where the patient is worried needlessly about the nurse because she is 15 minutes late.

- Always put specific directions to the client's home on the record so that finding the way will be easier for the nurse and other staff members who may visit the client.

# Discharge Planning

*Pat Carr, RN*

"Discharge planning begins the day the patient is admitted." As nurses working in home healthcare, we tend to view discharge planning as a hospital nursing responsibility. We frequently get annoyed if patients are discharged home and appropriate planning has not been done. It seems so obvious to us that discharge planning is important. What we sometimes forget is that we also discharge patients to another level of care and must assume responsibility for preparing our patients for independence. For us, as much as for anyone, discharge planning does begin the day the patient is admitted to our care.

At admission, we are concerned with what we can do for our patients. We plan our nursing activities, and we assure our patients that we will be there to help them. Sometimes we forget that the best way to help our patients is to plan all of our nursing activities with one eye firmly focused on patient independence. If we maintain that focus from the day of admission, we are planning for discharge with each visit.

Discharge planning is not a task isolated from all others. Planning for a patient's discharge is simply planning nursing procedures and instruction with the emphasis on patient independence. Table 1 shows several common problems in home health nursing. Two nursing interventions are shown: one with a strict nursing focus and the other with an emphasis on patient independence.

The list could go on and on. The point is, always keep the goal of patient independence in mind and plan nursing activities that will help the patient eventually function with confidence.

| TABLE 1. Nursing interventions for discharge planning | | |
| --- | --- | --- |
| **Problem** | **Nursing Focus** | **Patient Focus** |
| Patient confusion about medication administration | Set medications up weekly | Obtain medication dosage box and immediately begin instruction to family or neighbor |
| Need for weekly venipuncture for labwork | Nurse does all venipunctures | Nurse does first few venipunctures; checks with physician about decrease in frequency; immediately begins to make arrangements for transportation to lab when patient is able |
| Unstable CHF | Frequent visits for assessment | Visits as frequently as necessary, but also begin instructions regarding daily weights and signs and symptoms that the patient can identify and act on |

The patient who has been receiving care instruction throughout his or her nursing visits is much more prepared to assume responsibility for care when the time comes.

The concept is simple, but the application of the concept can be very difficult. After all, it is much easier for nurses to do "nurses things" than it is to modify those activities and teach the patient to do them. It is certainly easier to do a venipuncture every week that it is to teach the patient that eventually he or she will have to go to the laboratory, and plan for transportation when the time comes. We cannot take the easy way out. Patients get discharged for all reasons. When the time comes, the patient must be ready to assume responsibility. That readiness cannot be achieved by nursing instruction given on the last visit.

Discharge planning does begin at admission. It begins with careful patient instruction and the attitude that the patient will be able to care for himself or herself at some point. It also includes using nursing judgement and conferences with the physician to modify procedures so that they may be done by the patient, and making efforts to involve family and neighbors when necessary. The nurse's job is to do everything he or she can to move the patient toward independence. We have to do that job so well with each patient that we eventually are no longer needed. Hospitals may discharge patients home with home healthcare to share the responsibility, but we discharge our patients to themselves, their families, and the community. We have to prepare our patients for that outcome, and we have to do it right from the beginning.

# Two Halves Don't Make a Whole

*Patricia Carr, RN*

Published in *RN* July 1990.
Copyright 1990 Medical Economics Publishing.
Montvale, NJ. Reprinted by permission.

I worked in hospitals for a long time. I always thought I was doing a good job. I cared about my patients, worked hard to teach them to care for themselves, and felt good about the whole nursing process. When it came time for someone to go home, I would review the discharge instructions, wish him well, and turn my attention to the next patient.

Now I know that I was only doing half the job. As a home health nurse, which is what I am now, I do the other half. We nurses can't claim to give complete patient care until we've built a bridge between the two halves.

John needed that bridge. Hospitalized for two months with bacteremia and renal failure, he went home to a two-room apartment severely debilitated. The diet that his hospital nurse and dietitians had so painstakingly taught him was impossible to follow with only a hot plate and a small refrigerator, and he could not afford to fill his prescription.

It took weeks to get John's diet and medication orders altered to fit his resources. That meant valuable time lost toward recovery. The hospital nurse did her job and I did mine, but the discharge planning that should have connected us wasn't there.

Anna also fell into the gap between our two halves. Diagnosed as having an inoperable malignancy, she'd been hospitalized to have a permanent gastrostomy tube inserted in preparation for a course of outpatient radiation therapy. The hospital nurses did a wonderful job of teaching Anna how to care for her tube and use it for feeding.

What they didn't realize was that Anna had no way of getting to radiation therapy every day. And just as John could not afford his prescribed medication, Anna couldn't afford the liquid nutritional supplement ordered for her.

As Anna's home health nurse, I found transportation for her and got orders to substitute an affordable nutritional supplement that was available through a charitable organization. But this took time. Anna's therapy was delayed, and her nutritional status declined.

Compete care for Anna and John and dozens of other patients — especially those with no family to help them — requires personal discharge planning. Although there are some institutions that have an active social service department or a discharge planning nurse who coordinates many details, this is not often the case.

It falls then, to hospital nurses to look ahead and ask questions about finances and support systems. They need to be aware of the cost of prescriptions, limitations in the patient's home environment, and the availability of community resources.

On the home health side, I must assess the patient's needs before he's discharged, and plan care accordingly. My responsibility is to look for obstacles to good care and work with the family and hospital team to get around those obstacles before they interrupt the continuity of care.

Anna and John both returned to the hospital with complications of their diseases. They went with detailed transfer forms that spelled out the problems in their home care. For both of them, the second hospital discharge was smoother. The hospital and the home health agency were able to work together to bridge the gap between in-patient and home care.

I'd like to think that we can build a solid bridge that every patient can cross safely. Then, and only then, will we be able to say that we're doing a complete job for our patients.

# Evaluation of the Therapeutic Nurse-Patient Relationship

*Marshelle Thobaben, RN, MS, FNP*

Therapeutic interactions between the patient and the nurse provide the framework for the development of the therapeutic nurse-patient relationship. It forms the basis for the hallmark of nursing practice, which is caring. Recently I reviewed a home healthcare policy for screening the competency level of newly hired nurses. I was disappointed that the "check list" only included technical skills (i.e., start an I.V., do a sterile dressing). When I questioned the Director of Nurses as to the rationale for not including the nurse's ability to develop a therapeutic relationship as one of the basic competencies, she responded that the supervisors wanted to protect the patient's safety by evaluating the nurse's ability to perform technical skills. She assumed that nurses could communicate effectively with patients and that it was too difficult to evaluate their effectiveness at developing therapeutic relationships. I expressed my concern that by only including technical skills on the "check list" that the newly hired nurses would think the agency primarily valued their ability to be a technical nurse. In home healthcare, the nurse is often the only professional visiting the patient. This demands that nurses be exceptionally skilled in developing therapeutic relationships with patients so they are able to understand and be responsive to their patients' needs. It is a skill that needs to be evaluated when new nurses are hired and during all nurses' yearly evaluations.

An evaluation of a nurse's ability to develop therapeutic relationships with patients can be divided into two sections. First, is the nurse successful at interviewing patients? Second, does the is the nurse successful at interviewing patients? Second, does the nurse have the ability to achieve and maintain a relationship with patients successfully?

The first area of the nurse's evaluation is his or her ability to interview clients appropriately. Interviews can be formal or the information can be obtained from the patients while the nurse is performing other tasks. The ability to communicate effectively with clients is the basis of successfully interviewing clients. Evaluating a nurse's communication skills can be complex. The nurse could use therapeutic communication techniques, but still not be effective with the client interview because he or she did not develop a trusting relationship with the client. The evaluation would have to incorporate both the nurse's ability to use therapeutic techniques and to establish a trusting relationship with the client. Many communication techniques or approaches have proved to be effective in facilitating communication. There are several examples. The nurse can use open-ended, generalized, leading questions; state observations that are perceived about the patient; reflect, validate, or restate what the patient has said. The nurse can give feedback or summarize the main ideas with the patient; or the nurse can use silence thoughtfully to encourage the patient to talk and organize his or her thoughts.

Other approaches and techniques have proved to be barriers to therapeutic communication with patients. Examples include giving false reassurance, using cliches or stereotyped responses, being too strongly opinionated, using the wrong vocabulary, expressing either unnecessary approval or disapproval, agreeing or disagreeing with the patient, becoming defensive, changing the topic, bombarding the patient with questions, rejecting or belittling the patient, giving advice, stating personal experiences or opinions, or making value judgements.

The following list of questions could be used as a guide in an evaluation of a nurse's success in interviewing clients and using therapeutic communications skills.

- Does the nurse primarily use therapeutic responses that facilitate communication?
- Is the nurse aware of the barriers to effective communication he or she might be using?
- Does the nurse listen to what the patient is saying, verbally and nonverbally?
- Does the nurse communicate with the patient about the patient, and the patient's feelings, not about him or herself, other

patients, or the staff?
* Does the nurse indicate an awareness of cultural differences and avoid preconceived ideas, prejudices, biases, or imposing personal values on patients?
* Does the nurse respect confidentiality and only share patient information appropriately and when necessary with health team members?
* Does the nurse obtain the data needed to formulate a plan of treatment?
* Does the nurse evaluate his or her own ability to interview patients successfully?

The second area of evaluation is the nurse's ability to develop and maintain therapeutic relationships with patients. Therapeutic interaction between the patient and the nurse provides the framework for the development of the therapeutic nurse-patient relationship. During the introductory phase of the nurse-patient relationship, the foundation of the relationship is developed. It is the most crucial phase. The nurse is expected to establish a rapport with a patient, gain mutual trust, explain the purpose and the limitations of the home visits, clarify the patient's expectations of the relationship and the services, and begin the initial patient discharge plan. If a home healthcare nurse is not able to develop successfully a trusting relationship with his or her patient and have a mutually accepted plan of care, he or she will have difficulty with the case.

During the working phase of the nurse-patient relationship, the goals developed with the patient are addressed and evaluated as new data emerges. The nurse serves as an agent for the patient, supporting what is reasonable for the patient to achieve during the limited time frame of their relationship.

The termination is the final phase of the therapeutic nurse-patient relationship. The nurse prepares the patient for this phase throughout the relationship. The discharge date is generally known when the plan of treatment (POT) is developed with the patient. The POT includes the time frame during which the patient's goals are expected to be achieved. The plan's information helps the patient understand the home healthcare services to be provided and to be prepared for discharge. Before the patient's discharge, the nurse and the patient should evaluate the appropriateness and effectiveness of the POT.

An evaluation of a nurse's success in establishing a therapeutic relationship with clients could include the following questions.

- Does the nurse introduce himself or herself to clients?
- Does he or she explain the role of the home healthcare nurse?
- Does the nurse establish a trusting relationship with clients?
- Does he or she obtain the client's perception of his or her problems and what the client expects to gain from the services?
- Is the client included in establishing his or her goals for treatment?
- Is the client included when the goals for treatment are changed or met?
- Are the client's expectations regarding the services the agency will provide clarified?
- Does the nurse explain the time frame during which the services will be provided?
- Are appropriate referrals to other community resources made before the patient is discharged?
- Does the nurse terminate the services with the patient by having the patient evaluate the process and the usefulness of the services?

Newly hired and other home healthcare nurses should be evaluated for their ability to develop and maintain therapeutic relationships with their patients. Ensuring that home healthcare nurses have this competency will increase overall quality of the home healthcare agency services and improve consumer relations. Evaluation of the nursing staff will help them improve the quality of their practice and increase their awareness of the significance of therapeutic relationships. And finally in-service programs can be developed to address staff needs as identified by the evaluation process.

# The Home Care Nurse as Case Manager

*Linda Esposito, MPH*

Reproduced by permission of the National Association for Home Care,
From *Caring* magazine, Vol XIII, No 4, pp. 30-33.
Not for further reproduction.

As health care costs continue to rise and patients continue to enter home care with more acute situations, a gap grows between the homebound patient and access to health care. To bridge this gap the role of the home care nurse is evolving to encompass case management. Combined with personal care, case management helps the patient achieve his or her maximum health potential.

Managing 25 or more patients in a caseload can be extremely stressful, however, and there are few contemporary guidelines that describe how to manage a patient's and family's physical, emotional, and social needs (see Table 1). Successful case management means the home care nurse treats the family as a whole instead of isolating the treatment to the patient. Often the primary goal is independence for patient and family, but if this is not possible the home care nurse assists in mobilizing the needed resources.

Following are 10 steps through which nurses pass in home care case management. These steps are a continuum; some steps may be repeated, the order may vary, and some steps may not apply in every case. They may be used as a guideline to help the home care nurse formulate his or her own style in case management.

## STEP ONE: INITIAL REFERRAL AND ORDERS

Smooth admission to home services is vital to further management. The nurse must review the referral and orders to prepare for the first home visit. He or she should use information from the referral and orders to organize educational materials and required equipment for the patient and family.

## STEP TWO: THE FIRST HOME VISIT

The initial home visit is crucial in more than one respect. This visit helps build trust between the patient, family, and nurse. The nurse needs to assess the patient's financial and social systems as well as health. With the patient and family the nurse prioritizes the problems. Medications are evaluated by referencing them to the initial orders, looking at the actual bottles, and noting the patient's over-the-counter medication use. The nurse needs to assess the patient's and family's knowledge of medication administration and procedures and determine who is the main caregiver so the nurse can discuss future concerns, questions, and treatment changes. Instructions given to the patient and family must be written clearly and simply. Education sessions should last no longer than 20 minutes on the first home visit because both patient and family are usually stressed. The subsequent visit schedule will be determined at this first visit.

---

**Table 1. Tips on Scheduling a Caseload**

- Avoid scheduling more than two involved cases in one day. Mix each day's cases with home care aide supervision, Medicaid patients, and Medicare maintenance patients.
- Avoid overloading the patient and family with lengthy visits. Education sessions should last no longer than 20-30 minutes for optimal learning.
- Take travel time into consideration when scheduling patients, but remember that patient needs are the priority.
- When making the initial admission phone call, advise the patient and family that insurance cards, medication bottles, and any discharge instructions or papers from the hospital will be needed at the time of your visit.
- Try to make all followup phone calls to the physician, equipment company, or other providers from the patient's home at the time of your visit.
- Review the record and orders prior to each visit.
- Attempt to contact key family members to obtain their input and to give an update on the patient's condition and needs.
- Arrange team conferences on difficult cases.
- Try to complete documentation in the car or soon after the visit. This helps in recording the details of the visit.

---

The nurse evaluates whether the family or patient requires additional services such as therapy, social services, and home care aide assistance. It is the nurse's responsibility to instruct the patient and family on the roles of the other team members to guide decisions about further services. Discharge planning also begins at the first home visit by determining the treatment goals for the patient and family.

### STEP THREE:  COLLABORATING WITH TEAM MEMBERS

The nurse then consults with the referring physician and any other practitioners involved in the case. The nurse and physician collaborate to identify the patient's needs and problems. The nurse then changes or generates orders in accordance with the patient's response to treatment and need for additional services. Referrals are sent to other services. The nurse gives a report to each service involved in the case.

Communication between the nurse, physician, and other team members must be consistent. All team members need to be aware of the patient's response to treatment and whether any new problems arise. Most agencies encourage conferences at least once a week with the team members and the nurse coordinating the care. Communication also is encouraged as needed and can take the form of direct supervision during a home care visit, telephone contact, or team meetings, if necessary.

### STEP FOUR:  FORMULATING THE PLAN OF CARE

Once the problems have been identified with the input of the patient, family, nurse, physician, and other providers, the team can develop the plan of care. Most plans of care list the problem, short- and long-term goals, and the interventions needed to meet these goals.

Short- and long-term goals need to be written as measurable objectives. For example, a short-term goal might be that the patient and family will give a return demonstration of three signs and symptoms of congestive heart failure.

### STEP FIVE:  EVALUATING THE PLAN OF CARE

On each visit the nurse evaluates the plan of care and determines whether the interventions are helping the patient meet the established goals. The nurse also evaluates the goals themselves and adjusts them according to the patient's needs.

Goals established in the beginning of care may have been either unrealistic or too simple. The evaluation phase of the nursing process is a continuum and is important whenever there is contact with the patient. It is more effective for the team members to collaborate and discuss the patient's status in terms of established goals.

## STEP SIX:  ASSESSING NEW OR CHANGED NEEDS

During the visit the nurse evaluates the patient for new or changed problems and notifies the physician in the event of a change.   Services and medications may be added or cut as necessary. The nurse sends a short order form to the physician to verify the verbal orders.

Documenting any problems, action, and physician contact is extremely important.  It enhances the nursing process and helps ensure reimbursement.   Records should reflect the patient's progress and response to treatment. Successful, comprehensive documentation indicates the patient's condition and response to treatment, followup of any problems, nurse action, and the family's involvement in care.

## STEP SEVEN:  PREPARING FOR DISCHARGE

Discharge planning begins at the initial visit and continues with subsequent visits.   As the patient progresses the nurse will frequently assess the patient's goals and determine whether the patient and family have the ability to care for the patient. Services should be cut back slowly to assess the patient's and family's ability to provide care. For example the number of home care aide visits can be cut as the patient progresses.

Service is decreased only when the patient and family can begin caring for the patient safely. If the patient reaches a plateau and chronic needs exist, the nurse must educate the patient and family in how to obtain the needed resources.

Documentation must reflect the family's and patient's knowledge of the decrease of services, how they are going to function with this decrease, and how the nurse evaluates their response to the decrease on subsequent visits.

## STEP EIGHT:  EVALUATING FOR DISCHARGE

Once a patient has reached his or her maximum benefit from home care the nurse assesses the patient's and family's readiness for discharge by consulting with other team members involved in the patient's care.

## STEP NINE: REVIEWING THE RECORD

The nurse then reviews the record with the patient and family to go over the set goals and evaluation of the patient outcomes.

## STEP TEN: DISCHARGE

The patient and family should be well prepared to provide care independently on discharge. Ideally they should agree to the discharge and know whom to call if they have problems, the private resources available to them, and what community or state programs for which they are eligible.

The nurse records that all goals have been addressed and orders are complete; he or she then writes a discharge summary to reflect the care that was given.

# CHAPTER 4

# Patient Education

# Successful Client Teaching - What Makes the Difference?

*Janice Crist, RN, MS*

The setting where we perform our special type of nursing creates a unique challenge in patient education. Clients at home are in a more powerful position than patients in the hospital setting. They decide if they are going to follow through with our plan of treatment and teaching — whether it concerns a psychomotor skill such as insulin injections or changing a health habit such as quitting smoking.

What are our goals when we teach a client — compliance or presenting facts clearly enough to enable the client to make an informed decision? The art of patient education lies somewhere between — where we "facilitate" a behavior change. Let's examine these three approaches.

## WORKING TOWARD COMPLIANCE

We all try to achieve compliance when a behavior change is, in our view, vital to the client's health. Also, since compliance is a measurable goal, it fits nicely into the nursing diagnosis mode of care planning. With this approach, we may either use subtle coercion or be didactic. You and I know that although attempting to secure compliance may be the most direct form of teaching, we often receive lip service that yes, our client will comply, and then the teaching is ignored. Since the client does not "own" the learning goals we have set, he may have little motivation to comply.

Compliance connotes a scenario in which the patient passively obeys rules set down by the "boss" — in this case, you, the nurse. This medical model approach is one reason why I left hospital nursing. I prefer the educational model which encourages client autonomy and the ability to set learning goals. Motivational and self-care theory encourage this more active role for the client. However, let's not go to the opposite extreme, either.

## THE INFORMED DECISION APPROACH

This approach has 1970s "me generation" ring to it. It says, "Give the client the information; he can then decide whether or not to heed our recommendations." With this approach, we don't have to invest much time in establishing rapport before explaining the logic of using sterile technique on a dressing change, observing the patient practice the skill, or reinforcing our teaching with technically correct handouts and pictures. This approach is easy to use; it's direct, and if there is no follow-through, we do not have to feel that we failed. The client made the decision.

## THE FACILITATOR

Somewhere between these two approaches lies facilitating health behavior changes. In this role the nurse assists the client — who is the focus of the health care team and is responsible for his own self-care — to make the changes that he himself wants. There's no formula for using this approach. As a facilitator, I use my intuition on how to approach the client and use my "self" a lot in teaching. Both of these initiatives are important in establishing rapport as are the following:

*Listening.* Listen to the client's objections to change. The client may object to the fact that an acute myocardial infarction has occurred. You won't get him to quit smoking during his denial stage. As we learned from Kubler-Ross, we can't push someone into the stage of acceptance of a loss. Validating the feelings of the client is expressing — letting him know you understand his feelings: outrage, disbelief, loss of self-image — is the best way to help him move closer to acceptance. Then he is ready to learn.

*Clarifying.* I realized that a woman to whom I was teaching diabetes care was having trouble concentrating. I learned that she was worrying about her diet. She believed she would have to quit eating the foods she was used to. Once I understood she thought she would have to make a bigger life-style change than was really necessary, I explained that she could continue to eat most of her favorite foods, so long as she took care to measure and balance them throughout the day.

*Counseling with the family.* Get family members to discuss their feelings about the changes they and the client will have to make. Above all else, have the client and family discuss with one another what they feel about these issues. Promote the team spirit and include the family in your teaching. This team is a great reinforcer of your teaching. Also, families can help brainstorm on how to make changes fit realistically into the client's life-style.

*Being a role model.* Do you take care of yourself? Do you smoke? Are you overweight? Do you have lots of stress which is not balanced by play or relaxation? Clients can sense your nonverbal level of commitment to taking care of yourself. Clients are less motivated when the nurse-educator does not practice what she preaches.

You can probably recall cases in which your teaching was successful; examine the methods you used in those cases. You may be aware that you somehow helped (facilitated) those clients to achieve their learning goals.

Remember that although our clients have the power to choose their health behavior in the home setting, we can successfully facilitate patient education when we let them tell us what they feel about their illnesses and what they view as important to learn. Don't preach or merely give information; use your personal communication skills.

# Helping Older Learners Learn

*Jane Marie Crosbie, RN C, MS*

"I am so frustrated. I feel like giving up sometimes. I've been working with Mrs. Clayton for several weeks now and she seems absolutely unwilling to learn anything about diabetes or to even try to give herself her insulin. She lives alone, is fiercely independent, and is getting really annoyed at the idea that her daughter has to come by twice a day to give the injections for her. What is going on?"

This conversation with a new home health nurse led to my consultation with Mrs. Clayton, a pleasant 72-year-old woman, recently diagnosed as an insulin-dependent diabetic, and now labeled as noncompliant.

As I reviewed her records, I learned that Mrs. Clayton is a retired florist from North Carolina who has been widowed for 5 years. She recently moved to California to be near her daughter and grandchildren, and lives simply in a small garden apartment in the company of her dear pet, a tabby cat named Troubles. Financially, she gets by frugally with some savings and her social security income. She has few friends but seems to enjoy her reclusive lifestyle.

In addition to her diabetes, she has a medical history of osteoarthritis, chronic obstructive pulmonary disease, and hypertension. Except for some mild memory loss, she has no apparent cognitive deficits and is of above average intelligence. She has minor mobility problems that are related to arthritic pain, and tires easily, but is still able to devote time to her garden each week and cook her own meals.

Mrs. Clayton led me into her home, and was preparing tea for us as I questioned her about her colorful flowers. I noticed that when her back as turned to me, she did not respond to my comments. I also found it a little unusual that she wore no glasses and there were no reading materials of any kind in her small living-dining room.

When it seemed appropriate to discuss her sensory status, several things came to light. She said that she had a bit of trouble hearing, and although she normally wore a hearing aid, she had not been able to get to the drugstore recently for fresh batteries. She relied on lip reading to communicate in the interim. She had misplaced her glasses some time ago and could not afford new ones. She then added, "You know, I was embarrassed to tell my nurse that I couldn't see the little marks on those insulin syringes."

Over our second cup of tea, Mrs. Clayton emphatically stated that she just "couldn't believe" she was a diabetic at this late date. Her mother had also had diabetes, had suffered an amputation of her left leg, and had become totally dependent before her death from complications.

Sensory losses, financial constraints, denial, and fear of dependency are just a few of the barriers that had prevented Mrs. Clayton from learning about her disease. What a difference it would have made if her nurse had based her interventions on aging concepts.

## TEACHING AND THE AGED

The nature of our health care delivery system, coupled with the dramatic increase in our aging population, has created multiple needs for home teaching of the elderly.

With the advent of DRGs, the acutely ill aged convalesce at home and most often attend to unfamiliar procedures and equipment between nursing visits. Parenteral nutrition, sterile dressing changes, and personal comfort measures are areas that may need to be addressed.

On the other end of the acuity scale, a growing network of community services is giving more frail, dependent, and cognitively impaired elderly the opportunity to remain in the home setting, as opposed to institutionalization. Here, teaching comes in again: accident prevention, management of chronic disease, and rehabilitation techniques are but a few of the topics patients and caregivers may need to learn about.

Combining knowledge of adult learning theory with the principles of aging can result in positive health outcomes for both these groups of elders. An overview of concepts basic to gerontology will put some of the essentials into perspective as we consider the question: What makes teaching the older learner different from teaching the younger adult? Promoting independence and the highest level of wellness possible is the focus of gerontological nursing. It calls for a holistic approach because of the complex nature of normal age-related changes, the presence of chronic diseases, and the emotional, social, and functional losses that commonly accumulate with aging. The special needs of the aged are associated with the interrelationships among these issues, the uniqueness of the aging process for each person, and the individual's ability to adapt.[1]

In general, there is a decline in verbal and physical response time, a loss of reserve capacity to withstand stress, and progressive physiological degeneration. Despite the challenges and multiplicity of changes that come with advanced age, most older adults cope surprisingly well. Thorough assessments are vital to individualize teaching approaches and overcome age stereotyping.

## ATTITUDES AND VALUES

Learning is possible and desirable throughout the late stages of life. Although with normal aging, short-term memory, assimilation, and response time may be slowed, it is important to recognize that some elderly will perform as well as the young.[2] The nurse's attitude is critical. It is important to focus on patient strengths and expect the elderly to learn. My confidence in Mrs. Clayton's abilities very likely enhanced her self-esteem and alleviated some of the anxiety fostered by our culture and its negative attitudes toward the aged learner.

Independence and good health are of such significance to the aged that, ironically, these values may be barriers to learning. Changing health behaviors or learning new techniques may be threatening if viewed as "proof" that the individual has a condition that could lead to dependency. Being confronted with new information may also disrupt long-held beliefs and health habits.[3] Denial and anger can be dealt with by establishing trust, providing emotional support, and identifying specific fears. In Mrs. Clayton's case, discussing her fear of diabetes and its association with her mother's dependency and death was the first step toward collaboration in setting teaching-learning goals, a primary consideration when working with the aged and their families.[1]

## PHYSICAL CHANGES AND ENVIRONMENTAL ADAPTATIONS

A variety of physiological factors may also interfere with learning. With normal aging, sensory losses almost always occur. Visual changes include decreases in acuity and sensitivity to light, increased sensitivity to glare, and altered color vision.

For Mrs. Clayton, our first task was to get her a new pair of eyeglasses. A referral to the senior center's case management program was instrumental in arranging the funding and transportation to reach this goal. As Mrs. Clayton and I continued our visits, I sometimes needed to remind her to wear her glasses and clear off the smudges. She found that she could see much better. Her vision was further improved when we turned on a few extra room lights and adjusted the blinds to prevent window glare.

While teaching her the specifics about diabetes, I used large-print materials and diagrams in strong contrasting colors of red, orange, and yellow against a neutral background. Though not necessary for Mrs. Clayton, some clients with visual impairments also benefit from audiotapes, which can be left in the home for review.[2,4]

Hearing losses can also profoundly affect the older adult's ability to learn, especially since many will deny hearing problems, and, like Mrs. Clayton, rely mainly on lip reading to communicate. It is crucial that the home health nurse encourage the use of hearing aids and other adaptive hearing devices for those who find them beneficial.

After we carefully examined her budget, Mrs. Clayton decided to purchase a regular supply of hearing aid batteries when they went on sale every few months at a nearby discount store. Now that she could see better with her new glasses, she was able to handle her small hearing aid more easily and began inserting it most mornings before breakfast.

We were by then communicating much more effectively, but I found I could help her even more by positioning myself so that the light fell on my face as I spoke, speaking slowly and distinctly in a normal tone of voice, and checking with her frequently to make sure she was following me. Though Mrs. Clayton's home was quiet, I was aware that had her household been busy, I would have closed doors and turned off the television to decrease the background noises that could have distracted her.

In addition to being aware of sensory losses, it is important to recognize potential problems with the fatigue and pain often accompanying chronic disease and aging. For example, we scheduled Mrs. Clayton's sessions for mid-mornings, the most energetic part of her day. It was also helpful for her to take an ibuprofen tablet for her arthritic pain about an hour before our visit. I made sure that she was positioned comfortably in her favorite chair and that the room temperature was to her liking. Finally, I limited the teaching to 30- to 45-minute time increments to avoid undue stress and fatigue. These interventions seemed to work, since she remained alert and involved throughout her lessons.

## THE TEACHING PROCESS

As learning needs are assessed and collaborative goals realized, it is desirable to teach first what clients most want to know about the subject. Mrs. Clayton wanted to learn to give her own injections, was anxious to know if anything could be done so that she "wouldn't lose a leg like my mother," and was curious about the long-term effects the disease would have on her health and independence. We concentrated on only one aspect of these topics each visit, with short-term, easily attainable goals. This provided a climate of success and helped alleviate some of the cautiousness she felt toward learning. I also left written material she could review before our next session, to increase her confidence through advance preparation.

When pacing the lessons, I was mindful of the shortened attention span and additional time required for most elders to process information. I repeated and summarized points periodically, while encouraging her to ask questions or to repeat immediately the psychomotor procedures I had demonstrated. I also related each task to her overall goal for independence in order to make it more meaningful, but I avoided introducing extraneous ideas, which might have confused her.

Declining physical dexterity can be a problem for the old. Despite her new glasses and temporary relief from the arthritic pain in her hands, Mrs. Clayton still had some difficulty manipulating the syringes and medication vials. Since I anticipated that this might be a problem, I was able to be patient, use appropriate humor, and offer her sincere praise along the way. To facilitate her retention and recall, I left a hand-out with diagrams depicting each step of the procedure we had discussed. I also gave her our agency telephone number in case she had further questions or needed reassurance. During subsequent visits I reviewed the points we had previously covered in order to clarify any misunderstandings.

A final and very important part of the teaching process is to include family members when possible. Although Mrs. Clayton's daughter had been involved in her mother's care, she actually knew very little about her mother's condition or what to expect in the future. Luckily, she was able to make arrangements to attend some of our sessions, both for her own learning and to provide support and encouragement to her mother.

## RESISTANT LEARNERS

For a variety of reasons, some patients and families will be much more difficult to teach than Mrs. Clayton. There may be subtle cognitive impairments, unfinished grief work, or other cultural or emotional issues as yet unknown to the nurse. Sometimes the health changes called for may be too costly in terms of patient autonomy and family lifestyle. It is important to continue to assess, offer support, and recognize that, in the end, decisions rest with the client. This right must be respected. If safe care cannot be provided in the home, however, alternate strategies will have to be devised. Interdisciplinary referrals may be in order.

As to what became of Mrs. Clayton, she gradually came to accept her diabetes, and learned quite a bit about the disease, her dietary needs, and measures to prevent complications. She feels fortunate to be able to administer her own insulin injections and enjoys her relationship with her daughter much more now that she has regained her independence.

Working with the elderly is complex, challenging and enormously rewarding. Competent teaching by the home health nurse empowers the aged, helps prevent premature institutionalization, and enhances the health status and quality of life for older adults and their families.

---

**REFERENCES**

1. American Nurses' Association. *Standard of Gerontological Nursing Practice.* Kansas City, Mo, American Nurses' Association, 1976.
2. Kim KK. Patient education. In: Burggraf V, Stanley M eds. *Nursing the Elderly: A Care Plan Approach.* Philadelphia, JB Lippincott, 1989, 36-40.
3. Yurick AG, Spier BE, Robb SS, et al. *The Aged Person and the Nursing Process,* 3rd. ed. Norwalk, Conn., Appleton & Lange, 1989, 384-388.
4. Elioupoulos C. *A Guide to the Nursing of the Aging.* Baltimore, Williams & Wilkins, 1987, 34, 216-218.[1]

# Patient Education: Motivating the Learner

*Marjorie McHann, RN, BS*

Patient and family education is very important to promote quality, cost-effective patient care. Accreditation, reimbursement, and professional nursing organizations all recognize patient education as a key component of quality patient care. As a home health nurse, it's imperative for you to have a working knowledge of the teaching-learning process and be able to implement it with patients and families in the home setting.

A very important learning principle is that motivation is necessary for learning to occur. In fact, motivating the learner is often the crucial point in teaching. Following are some specific ways to enhance motivation and learning for your home health patients.

*Develop a good rapport with the patient and his family.* Even the family's dog should be acknowledged if he seems to be an important family member. Good rapport will not of itself guarantee successful teaching, but it does promote learning and is a factor that you can control to a large extent.

*Stress the patient's learning responsibility.* Tell the patient what you plan to teach and why. Let him know what part you expect him to play in the learning process. For instance, you might say to a diabetic patient: "After our discussion today you should be able to describe the 3 elements of diabetes treatment and explain how each helps to control your body's blood sugar levels." Encouraging the patient's participation will go a long way toward promoting motivation.

*Start where the learner is.* New learning must be based on

previous knowledge and experience. For instance, understanding an ADA diet requires basic knowledge of nutrition and food groups. The point where you begin teaching will be determined by what the learner knows about nutrition and diet. Content that flows from the familiar to the unfamiliar promotes learning.

*Use your communication skills.* Present your message clearly and enthusiastically, using words that the patient can understand. Use analogies and illustrations to help clarify concepts. Incorporate audio-visual aides into your teaching to stimulate the patient's eyes as well as his ears, thereby improving retention. Ask questions and wait for answers. If communication flows in one direction only (from nurse to patient) he will remember little of what he hears.

*Don't forget to listen.* This is a very important communication skill. Listen to the patient's objections to change. Often he is feeling a loss and your listening helps validate the feelings he needs to express such as anger, disbelief, and loss of self-image and helps him move closer to acceptance, where he will be more ready to learn. Above all, don't contradict, deny the reality of fears, or offer useless platitudes, such as "everything will be alright," for these actions can block the learning process.

*Encourage participation.* Effective learning requires active participation. Simply stated, we learn by doing, and the "doing" may involve a variety of activities:

- perceiving through the sense organs
- carrying on physical actions
- using mental process

This involvement is essential for learning and the more thoroughly the patient participates, the more effective will be the learning. Your role is to provide opportunities for participation and to encourage the patient to take advantage of them.

*Make learning relevant.* A common problem is that the patient sees no reason for learning what the nurse wants to teach. Adults, especially, resist learning isolated facts and theory which is not applied to practical problems. However, learning is enhanced if the learning goals are congruent and relevant to the life needs of the patient.

*Provide feedback.* Praise your patient when he demonstrates mastery of the material. Positive reinforcement will motivate him to stay involved in the learning process. As he gains confidence, his own satisfaction may become the source of feedback. The fact that satisfaction reinforces learning is bound up closely with the concept of motivation.

In summary, no one can assure that even the most skillfully

executed teaching plan will reach a patient and motivate him to act. Sometimes confusion, denial, or the severity of illness will prevent your patient from absorbing even the most simple concepts. But in most cases, you'll find that, by applying the principles of teaching and learning, you'll enhance effective patient education. As a result, you'll maintain standards of quality care, promote better patient outcomes, and insure more cost-effective patient care.

# Health Teaching: The Crux of Home Care Nursing

*Karen Hellwig, RN C, MN*

Imagine yourself as a home care nurse visiting Ms B. Your hearty knock on the door brings Ms W., Ms B.'s caregiver, to welcome you. She leads you to a cheerfully decorated room inhabited by Ms B., a diabetic who has had a past cerebrovascular accident, is aphasic, is essentially paraplegic, and requires assistance with all activities of daily living. Ms B. smiles up at you from her hospital bed and utters an unintelligible greeting. On this initial visit you assess Ms B.'s needs through a physical examination and your interview with Ms W. Ms B. is diapered for incontinence and has a gastric tube in place with signs of inflammation at the insertion site.

*Crucial to your nursing treatment plan will be teaching Ms W. about this client's care.* First you will need to develop a teaching strategy that will lead to optimum health and prevent recurrence of problems. Several educational theories can give you direction in determining your teaching plan. Some of the most widely used theories include motivational, planned change, and learning. Table 1 illustrates how each of these theories could be applied to the scenario above.

*Once you have established your teaching strategy, you need to determine what you will teach.* As a home care nurse, you focus your instruction on filling in the gaps. The caregiver may already have a basic understanding of the problem and its treatment. You will need to provide her with more in-depth knowledge. You may need to teach her new skills such as wound care and blood glucose monitoring. You may need to provide her with information on

| Table 1.  Three Teaching Theories as Applied to Ms W. | | |
| --- | --- | --- |
| **Teaching Theory** | **Description** | **Application** |
| Motivational | Relate serious consequences and high chance of recurrence to the health problem as the incentive to learn | Point out to Ms W. the possible ramifications of the untreated infected gastrostomy site in an effort to motivate learning |
| Planned Change | Identify problem areas and involve learner in the process of solving the problems | Identify patient immobility as the problem and strategize with the learner such things as position change, range of motion, increasing fluids, and massage |
| Learning | Respond to learner uncertainty or frustration by initiating a behavior that is reinforced through reward | Respond to the learner's uncertainty about diabetes by initiating insulin administration, blood glucose monitoring, diet, etc., and reward learner participation with positive feedback |

dosage, medication action, side effects, and schedule. You may need to help your client learn coping strategies. At times you may need to clarify information or clear up misconceptions. Finally, you may need to help to modify attitudes, sometimes of the caregiver and sometimes of the patient.

*Knowing how to teach is just as important as knowing what to teach.* Having acquired a repertoire of educational theories to draw from and an understanding of what a home care nurse is expected to teach, you are ready to begin teaching. In Table 2, you will see teaching structured as a seven-step process that includes assessing the setting, assessing the learner, assessing the teacher, determining the content and setting goals, planning and implementing teaching strategies, evaluating and documenting.

Finally, here are some tips for teaching that can make you more successful and your client more comfortable:

1. Be sure that the information you plan to impart is meaningful to the learner.
2. Reinforce positive learning behaviors and encourage the learner to make his/her own decisions regarding the learning experience.
3. Promote a positive, comfortable learning environment, and

**Table 2. Seven Steps in the Teaching Process as Applied to Ms W.**

| Teaching Process | Teaching Strategies | Implementation |
|---|---|---|
| Assess the setting | Ensure environment is conducive to learning and consider appropriateness of the available resources | Turn off TV and limit distractions. Provide comfortable seating. Assemble equipment and pamphlets for demonstrations. |
| Assess the learner | Consider client/caregiver's age, education, motivation, etc., and what effect change will have on those involved | Use appropriate vocabulary. Pace yourself appropriately. Be sensitive to the learner's beliefs and values and how the caregiver and patient relate to each other. |
| Assess the teacher | Consider your own attitudes and feelings, and assess your knowledge and ability to handle the situation | Accept the learner for who he or she is. Review materials and procedures to be taught (eg, gastrostomy site care, diabetic diets, medications, and foot care). |
| Determine content and set goals | Establish attainable, measurable short- and long-term goals in conjunction with the learner | Ask such questions as, "What do you expect to get out of this?" Set measurable goals such as, "The caregiver will correctly state actions of all client medications." |
| Plan and implement strategies | Use a variety of methods and modalities to convey information and teach procedures | Provide reading material (eg, pamphlet on Accu-chek II, the blood glucose monitoring machine). Use modeling, coaching, and demonstrations to teach skills (eg, supervise Ms W. on gastrostomy site care). Relate information to experiences. Counsel and share personal experiences. |
| Evaluate your teaching | Assess whether goals were met, which techniques worked, and whether the learner is willing and prepared to effect change | Ask the learner for feedback (eg, can caregiver correctly state actions of patient's medications?). Support the learner in his or her decision whether to implement learning. |
| Document your teaching and the learner's learning | Document goal achievement and nonachievement, compliance and noncompliance | Document successful strategies (eg, Ms W. able to perform gastrostomy site care correctly; knowledge deficit re: use of blood glucose monitor). Document your actions and the client's response in your nurse's notes (eg, "Pt states she has not been taking meds in spite of instructions on action and importance of meds"). |

reduce the learner's level of anxiety through therapeutic communication skills.

4. Allow enough time for the teaching sessions, especially if the learner has a sensory or learning disability.
5. Encourage the learner to apply a new skill/information immediately — 55% of new learning is forgotten one hour later, 65% by the next day, and 75% in one week.
6. Teach in small doses.
7. Start slowly and proceed from the known to the unknown. Assess what the learner knows and fill in the gaps.
8. Involve all the senses as much as possible (e.g., malodor is a sign of infection).
9. Use repetition.
10. Allow the learner control in the learning situation and decrease the potential for manipulation as a ploy to satisfy such secondary gains as avoiding work or gaining attention.

The goal of health education is self-care — and care of the self in the home is what we strive for in home care nursing. Teaching strategies such as those outlined here will, it is hoped, assist you in your quest for maintaining your home care clients and families at their highest level of functioning.

# Needs to Know, Wants to Know, Ought to Know

*Pat Carr, RN*

Nurses in home health are always teaching. Unfortunately, patients are not always learning. For information to be transferred successfully from nurse to patient, there has to be real interest and enthusiasm on both sides. There has to be a middle ground between the nurse and the patient where both are comfortable. There are times when this territory is hard to find or slippery to stand on.

Finding the elusive middle ground can be made easier by planning and flexibility on the part of the nurse. Patient education can be broken down into three areas. The first is that information that the patient needs to know to maintain his or her safety. The second is the information the patient wants to know about his or her care, and the third is the information that the nurse wants the patient to know. Communication frequently breaks down when the nurse puts the third area ahead of the second.

The first area is vital to the patient's safety at home. Hospital stays are shorter than ever before, and patients are coming home in unstable conditions. They have to know how to take their medications correctly. They have to know how to recognize life-threatening complications, and they have to know what to do in an emergency. To determine exactly what information belongs in this teaching area, the home health nurse only has to consider what a particular patient may experience during his first few days at home.

Once emergency procedures, complications, and medications are covered, the nurse moves to the second area of teaching. This involves dealing with what the patient perceives as important to his or her care. There are pitfalls here for the nurse. The patient's questions may not seem important, or the nurse may feel that there are other areas of teaching that are more important. This is the time to remember that teaching is useless if the learner is not interested. The nurse may feel that knowing how to manage edema is a priority for the patient, while the patient would rather talk about diet. This is the time for compromise. The nurse can use the patient's interest, answer questions about diet, and guide the conversation to include information about edema.

Once the first two areas have been dealt with, the nurse is in a position to work on teaching whatever else the patient should know.  By this time, the patient's own concerns have been addressed, and he or she may be more receptive to learning new material.  The nurse may then complete the plan of teaching, knowing that an environment has been created where learning can take place.

Every patient is an individual, and a teaching plan must be flexible. Factors such as the patient's attention span, anxiety level, level of physical comfort, and the physical environment must be taken into consideration when a teaching plan is considered. The grouping of topics into *needs to know, wants to know, and ought to know* can form the framework for any teaching plan. By using these three groups, emergencies can be dealt with, the patient's concerns can be addressed promptly, and the nurse can convey the information he or she considers appropriate. Patient and nurse can get together on the middle ground where teaching and learning meet.

# CHAPTER 5

# Quality Assurance Issues

# Quality Assurance in Home Care Services

*Florence S.Y. Hughes, RN*

"Quality Assurance in Home Care Services," by Florence S.Y. Hughes
Reprinted with permission from *Nursing Management,*
Vol. 18, No. 12, December 1987 issue.

Quality care, quality assurance and assurance of excellence: these are key words found in the professional literature. However, journal articles on quality care and quality assurance are usually written from the professional's perspective, often neglecting the patient's point of view and patients' rights. The present paper attempts to incorporate the patient's perspective by focusing on the rights of patients and showing how consideration of these rights can help to improve the quality of home care agencies. A survey of patient or client concerns conducted by Jo-Ann Friedman provides the basis for many of the patient issues to be addressed.[1]

## HOME CARE SERVICES

Home health professionals provide care to patients at home under the supervision of a physician. Usually, nurses coordinate the care of patients, often with the assistance of social workers, respiratory therapists or other specialists. Nonprofessionals, like aides and housekeepers, assist the patient with household chores, baths, etc.[2]

Home care facilities have increased in numbers within the last decade because of several factors. One reason is that numerous hospitals are organizing their own home health agencies to provide continuity of care to their patients. This is needed especially by older and weaker patients.[3] In part, these changes have resulted from the 1982 amendment of the original Medicare legislation which initiated prospective payments, thus changing the entire reimbursement process to hospitals. Because of this law, patients are released sooner, and often are referred to home care or private duty nurses.[4]

Another reason for expansion of home care services throughout the nation is the continual advancement made in medical technology. Improved equipment and increasing technical skill have made possible the performance of highly complex treatments at home. These include chemotherapy, supplemental IV therapy, physical and occupational therapy, and various therapies for speech, respiratory, and renal problems.

According to Friedman's survey, the primary concerns of home care patients included: 1) whether the home care agencies were regulated by federal or state laws or commissions, 2) how the different types of home care services were rendered, 3) whether the staff personnel were qualified and 4) how regulations on safety measures were implemented in the home.

Some home care agencies are certified and accredited by federal and state commissions; most are accredited by Medicare and the Joint Commission on Accreditation of Hospitals (JCAH), which certifies home care agencies as having met certain standards of health care. JCAH requires the agency to monitor and evaluate patient care on a continual basis; this process is known as a quality assurance program. "This represents the professional perspective about the quality of health care."[2] In addition to this, however, it is important that the rights of the patient be incorporated into the quality assurance program in order to attain satisfactory results.


## PATIENTS' RIGHTS

Patients' rights are not inherent, but are derived from societal values. A claim for certain rights has validity within a social order and these rights must be recognized by the society. According to the National League for Nursing's "Patients' Bill of Rights," patients have rights to health care that is accessible and appropriate for their health needs.[5] In providing these health care services in the home, professionals such as nurses, doctors, physical therapists and others must protect these rights. People do not lose their rights just because of illness or disease.

Home care patients usually do not demand their rights but they do request consideration and respect; patients would like to be treated with dignity and kindness. Because nurses and other health care providers tend to be task oriented, frequently they fail to devote time and effort to developing warm relationships with clients. Yet, interpersonal relationships with the patients are essential since they are conducive to better outcomes. For example, faster recuperation lessens health care costs; increased motivation in learning enhances knowledge in self care. Better acceptance of a terminal diagnosis helps to prepare a patient for death.

One of the most inviolate of patients' rights in confidentiality. This should never be violated by the professionals who take care of the patient in the home. All information relating to treatment or care is privileged because of the patient-nurse relationship and must be held in trust. All patients' medical and social information, including data in computer storage, must be kept confidential.

If a patient's right to confidentiality is violated, he or she can seek legal redress, especially if there are monetary or other damages as a result. Medical information can be mentioned by a professional casually or in an inappropriate place, resulting in an employee's discharge from a job. This patient has grounds to file a suit against the professional to recover damages for loss of income and mental suffering.

The patient's right to safe health care in the home is equally important. The only essential difference between home and the hospital environment is the type of equipment used in the home and the people who provide the care at home. "High-tech" equipment, such as monitors, usually is not available in the home, and the nurse is there only a brief period. Most home care is provided by family and significant others since professionals may visit the home once a day or less.

Thus, the nurse or coordinator of services must involve everyone in the learning process. The nurse should teach the patient and responsible family members about the patient's medications and their side effects to assure against errors in administration. The nurse must caution about patient falls caused by side effects of medications such as antipruritics, tranquilizers, and sedatives. These medications have cumulative effects, especially in older or weaker patients subject to increased ataxia or disorientation. Delirious patients attempt to get out of bed, fall and can be injured seriously.

The nurse can implement measures to help make the home free from hazards, with the cooperation of patient and family. Home furnishings can be rearranged to lessen accidental injury to the patient and hand rails can be installed for assisting a patient's mobility within the home. Also, the nurse should educate the patient about personal safety, taking into consideration the patient's educational level in the process. Written instructions should be used to reinforce the nurse's teaching and to reassure and remind the patient if he forgets what to do.

Professionals not only should teach clients but also learn from them and their family. Through listening to patients and their families, nurses will learn about cultural differences and the way different people view illness and health practices. This information must be taken into account when planning a care program. Cultural sensitivity will enhance the quality of care rendered to patients.

Refusal of care is the patient's right. If he feels that the treatments or medications are not benefiting him, he can stop them and ask for alternatives. Of course, the physician must be informed and the patient must be told of the consequences of this decision. Nevertheless, patients are entitled to refuse treatment even if they have no apparent reason for doing so.[2] Occasionally, when patients refuse treatment because of traditional beliefs or unrealistic fears, a conscientious team of physician and nurse can persuade clients to accept the procedure by educating them about its benefits.

Another important patients' right is full information about diagnosis and prognosis after hospital discharge.[6] Usually, there is no hesitation when the news is good, but doctors find it difficult to communicate about serious disease with poor prognosis. When this happens, the nurse must collaborate with the physician to decide how patient and family should be informed. Through her contacts with the patient and family, the nurse can share her insights about their attitudes so the physician can act appropriately. When patient and family are not informed sufficiently, they may become confused and anxious; this can result in anger and lack of cooperation. Any situation can be managed better if everyone understands the condition and its prognosis.

## QUALITY ASSURANCE

Quality of care issues are particularly difficult to address in home health settings. There is no consensus among the home care agencies as to what constitutes quality in home care services.[4] Quality includes those distinguishing characteristics that determine the value, rank or degree of excellence. There can be objective aspects of quality, but it is also a subjective and relative value that people want in a service or product. Measuring quality of care in the home is less objective than in a hospital, as the determinants are hard to quantify and it cannot be controlled as readily. However, standards and criteria originating in the hospital are used to develop those applicable to home care.

Assuring the client a specified degree of quality in health services is accomplished through continuous measurement and evaluation of structural components. These may include goal directed nursing process and/or consumer outcome and employ preestablished criteria and standards as available norms.[7] A critical part of quality assurance is evaluation of interventions made to remedy existing deficiencies.

Quality in home care encompasses the entire health care agency: 1) the administrator, nurses and other professionals; 2) the policies and procedures, 3) accurate documentation and 4) a well-established communication system.

A well-planned, systematic and ongoing method of monitoring and evaluating is essential to a quality assurance program. To be effective, a comprehensive program has to include well-established criteria for standards on the structure and outcomes. Structure refers to agency logistics: personnel and material. Outcome refers to those established and measurable criteria for nursing care and results that have been pre-established and set by the staff of the agency.

The paperwork involved in adequate documentation may seem tedious, but it is very important for determining the quality of total health care provided to patients. Only when the patient reaches his goals and attains maximum use of his physical and mental faculties, and the professional has evaluated this progress as successful, is maximum quality of care achieved.[8]

Quality in the provision of home care improves when patients' rights are incorporated into the patient care plan. To guarantee that these rights will be protected requires that nurses be selected carefully and oriented to the home care program.

## STANDARDS OF CARE

Standards are acknowledged measures of comparison for quantitative or qualitative values. Since professional nurses usually are the coordinators of total care for patients, they use standards to determine whether care was acceptable, both to the profession and the patient. To determine the effectiveness and efficiency of the health care services, the nurse must use specific criteria and measurable parameters. These standards are formulated and improved using the four-step cyclic nursing process: assessment, planning, implementation, and evaluation.[9]

Generally, standards are important to any company which provides services and/or manufactures products. Just as social, environmental and technological changes lead to alterations in service and product standards, changes in standards and criteria must be made by nurses. Standards determining the quality of health care should be reviewed, monitored and evaluated continuously by quality control committees to enable nurses to keep pace with new developments in health care.

There are three types of standards in nursing: 1) standards of structures which consider the organizational framework; 2) standards of process which encompass the procedures in health care to patients and 3) standards of outcomes which consider the objectives or goals of patients.[10] All must be given equal weight and scrutinized with the same degree of diligence to assure quality of care.

Recognition of professional nurses' roles and patients' rights and perspectives can improve quality of care in home health care agencies. Home care nurses must be willing to reach a compromise with patients' wishes in order to make mutually satisfying decisions on attainable goals and objectives. Independent, decisive nurses can coordinate home services in such a way that both patients' satisfaction and the nurses' objectives are achieved. As most patients opt for health care at home rather than in hospital settings, they look to home care professionals for guidance and supportive assistance.

---

**REFERENCES**

1. Friedman, Jo-Ann, "Guiding Patients Through the Labyrinth of Home Health Care Services," *Nursing and Health Care,* June, 1986, p. 306.
2. Stuart-Sidall, Sandra, *Home Health Care Nursing,* (Rockville: Aspen Systems Corporation, 1986), p. 16.
3. Frasca, Cathy and Meg W. Christy, "Assuring Continuity of Care Through a Hospital-Based Home Health Agency," *QRB,* 1986, 12(5): 167-171.
4. Mundinger, Mary O'Neil, *Home Care Controversy,* (Rockville: Aspen Systems Corporation, 1983), p. 24.
5. Rowland, Howard S. and Beatrice L. Rowland, *Nursing Administration Handbook,* (Rockville: Aspen Systems Corporation, 1980), p. 139.
6. Pozgar, George D., *Legal Aspects of Health Care Administration,* (2nd Edition), (Rockville: Aspen Systems Corporation, 1983), p. 116.
7. Schmadl, John C., "Quality Assurance: Examination of the Concept," *Nursing Outlook,* July, 1969, pp. 462-465.
8. Daniels, Kaye, "Planning for Quality in the Home Care System," *QRB,* 12:7: 247-251.

9.  Nichols, Christine A. and Maryann B. Wirginis, "Linking Standards of Care with Nursing Quality Assurance — the SCORE Method," *QRB*, 11:2:57-63.
10. Meisenheimer, Claire Gavin, *Quality Assurance,* (Rockville: Aspen Systems Corporation, 1985), pp. 53-61.

# Patient Complaints

*E.A. Huebner*
*P.E. Harrison*

Reprinted from *The Home Care and Documentation Guide*
by E.A. Huebner and P.E. Harrison, pp. 12:2-3,
with permission of Aspen Publishers, Inc., © 1991.

One of the patient rights is the "right to voice grievances regarding treatment or care that is (or fails to be) furnished or regarding the lack of respect for property by anyone who is furnishing services on behalf of the home health agency and must not be subjected to discrimination or reprisal for doing so." OBRA 87. Patients have the right to complain about services that are being (or not being) provided, the right to complain about the way they or their belongings are being treated, and the right to do it without fear of repercussions. They have always had this right, but now agencies are required to inform patients formally of this right and to encourage them to voice any complaints they may have. Some patients have feared complaining because they worried that if they complained, they might lose services they desperately needed. Home health agencies must also tell patients about their state's home health hotline number, which they can call if their complaints are not successfully resolved by the agency. Agencies are also required to document complaints, as evidence of compliance with the COP.

It is now and always has been a good business practice to encourage patients to complain, since problems must be identified if they are to be resolved. In other words, "You can't fix it if you don't know it's broke." A patient's complaint may provide the impetus needed to implement a quality assurance activity to determine if the complaint is an isolated situation or an indicator of a more widespread problem. Concrete evidence and documentation of problems is often needed to substantiate that, indeed, a problem exists, and to initiate measures to manage the problem.

For example, a patient's complaint about having too many different nurses visiting may result in a review of the clinical record and scheduling a procedure, not only for that patient but for others as well. A problem with continuity of care could be identified here, one that could be successfully managed. An awareness of the problem could lead to an improved scheduling system and a quality assurance activity focused on monitoring continuity of care. These changes could result in fewer nurses visiting individual patients and improved continuity in the care provided. Other benefits may be improved risk management and increased nurse satisfaction with the job. There should be a decreased likelihood of mistakes made with improved continuity of care. This should lead to a decreased risk of malpractice or negligence litigation.

When continuity of care is not seen as a problem or monitored in any way, management may have no clear idea how many different nurses or aides are seeing individual patients over time. As they try to accommodate new patients, staff scheduling and emergency situations, it is easy for agency management to be unaware of problems in this area. Had the patient in the example not complained, this issue might not have been addressed by management.

Problems with continuity of care usually affect quality of care, patient satisfaction, and employee satisfaction. Home care practitioners usually like to get to know "their" patients and want to follow through with their teaching and care plans. Patients also usually like to get to know "their" nurse, aide, or other staff person, and feel more comfortable having services provided by the same staff members. This one complaint, if managed properly, could potentially lead to operational improvements that could have significant paybacks for the agency at a very low cost. Improving quality does not always mean spending a large amount of money.

Management and staff must recognize that only a small percentage of unsatisfied clients actually register complaints verbally and an even smaller percentage complain in writing. Therefore, every complaint must be treated seriously.

Complaints need to be handled in a professional manner to clearly identify the real problems. Patients and their family members need to feel that someone at the agency has really listened to their complaints and will assist them in resolution of the real or perceived problem. When patients and family members are treated with respect and have their complaints investigated and resolved, if possible, they usually become very loyal clients. When people are not satisfied with the way their complaints are handled, they usually tell several other people about their bad experience — which damages the agency's reputation.

Home health care is a difficult business to manage since visiting staff are in patients' homes and functioning independently. Supervision of staff is especially important and challenging. The home environment and all of the emotional responses to illness and disability can present a myriad of problems for all parties involved. Shortages of professional, and, in some parts of the country, ancillary personnel further complicate the situation.

Documentation should be maintained on all complaints received from patients, families, referral sources, and physicians. The date the complaint is received, along with the names of the patient involved must be documented. If someone other than the patient is registering the grievance, agency staff should ask for that individual's name, mailing address, and phone numbers (home and work) so the agency may contact them to follow up on the situation. The nature of the complaint and the names of any personnel involved (or a description of the staff member) should be ascertained and documented. The log can be used as a worksheet. Use as many lines as necessary to clearly describe the complaint, follow-up actions, and to add any comments.

Complaints should be thoroughly investigated by management personnel, and appropriate action should be taken. It is very important that staff not be accused of wrongdoing without a chance to present their side of the story. Following the investigation, follow-up contact should be made with the patient or person that registered the grievance to demonstrate the agency's commitment and its efforts to remedy the problem or to present additional information as appropriate. The Log of Complaints can be used to record information obtained while investigating the complaint and to record any follow-up actions. Keeping this information in an organized format will help follow up with concerned parties as well as help maintain preparedness for state surveys. Surveyors may ask for this information, looking for evidence that complaints are being encouraged and acted upon by the agency's management.

# Patient Satisfaction and Quality Assurance

*Marjorie McHann, RN, BS*

## WHY PROMOTE PATIENT SATISFACTION?

As you know, patient satisfaction is now considered an important outcome measure for quality of care for a home health agency.

First of all, the increasing consumer rights movement in the United States has focused a greater emphasis on quality assurance, resulting in keen competition between home health agencies. This increasing competition for patients has caused agencies to become more concerned about their patients' perceptions of the quality of their care. As nurses, we are in a pivotal position to promote agency public relations because of our close contact with patients, doctors and other health care professionals.

Second, satisfied patients are more likely to achieve a better clinical outcome than dissatisfied patients. The outcome of care depends largely upon patient and family attitudes, expectations, response to nursing interventions and satisfaction with other agency encounters. As nurses, we're in a crucial position to influence patients' perceptions and, consequently, their behavior during care. Whether it be responding to a phone call in a timely fashion or providing physical and emotional interventions in an unrushed, caring and supportive manner, attention by a professional nurse is one of the most therapeutic interventions a patient can receive. When these therapeutic interventions are managed appropriately, they improve patients' responses to other interventions. When they are mismanaged or left to chance, recovery can actually be delayed.

And third, patient satisfaction is recognized as an important indicator of quality care by reimbursement, accreditation and professional organizations alike:

- Medicare requires agencies to address patients' viewpoints with surveys, a patient bill of rights, and a state hotline number for quality of care concerns.
- For accreditation, JCAHO and CHAPS require agencies to monitor, evaluate and consider patient and caregiver satisfaction with services provided.
- ANA and NLN standards of nursing practice enjoin nurses to be sensitive to patients' feelings and responsive to their needs.

## WHAT PATIENTS EXPECT FROM NURSES

In the past, our priority was clinical competence. Today, patients <u>expect</u> competence. Now they equate quality with more personal care.

It's important to remember that patients' priorities can be a lot different from nurses' priorities. We may judge ourselves by how quickly we "cure" our patients, but they judge us on more than that. Specifically, patients judge us by:

- how courteous we are
- how quickly we respond to their needs
- how much time we spend with them
- our physical appearance
- our tone of voice, and
- our nonverbal communication.

Clearly what counts most in the patient's mind is the human element, what used to be called bedside manner. In fact, studies on customer service report that, more than anything else, people value care and concern. Most of the time that people (including patients) don't return a business, it's because they sensed disinterest; they felt ignored and that nobody cared. Of course, other factors besides nursing care affect patient satisfaction, but home health nurses are with the patients day in and day out, and they play a vital role in promoting patient satisfaction.

## NURSE BEHAVIORS THAT PROMOTE PATIENT SATISFACTION

*Be sure your patient and his caregiver receive adequate orientation to home care services.* Mr. Halifax was admitted to home care for skilled nursing services following hospitalization for acute congestive heart failure and cardiac arrhythmias. During the

---

**Issues related to the perception of quality and the rating of satisfaction of home health consumers.**

1. Predischarge preparation and instruction
2. Orientation of patient/caregiver to home health services
3. "Styles of care" mean the most
4. Scheduling and timing of visits
5. Continuity of direct care staff
6. Staff attire
7. Concern, listening, attention
8. Teaching appropriate to learning readiness, education and ethnicity
9. Preserving patient dignity and privacy
10. Patient/caregiver perception of outcome and preparation for discharge from home care

---

Source: Adapted from "Home Care Consumers Speak Out on Quality" by Mary Lou V. Stricklin, MSN, RN, MBA. **Home Healthcare Nurse,** Volume 11, Number 6.

---

first visit, Mr. Halifax's nurse took the time to speak slowly, use simple language and repeat important instructions. She gave clear instructions about how to reach the nurse in an emergency, and she provided instructional materials about his heart condition and dietary requirements. As a result, Mr. Halifax and his wife felt less apprehensive and better able to respond positively to her nursing interventions.

*Use effective verbal and nonverbal communication skills to establish and maintain a good rapport with the patient and his family.* Mr. Halifax's nurse was careful to be sure her body language, tone of voice and words were consistent, and that they communicated sincerity and concern for the patient and his wife. A good relationship between the nurse and Mr. and Mrs. Halifax helped establish trust, contribute to improved compliance with the treatment plan, and promote better patient outcomes.

*Provide good customer service.* It's important to make the patient and family feel good about the service they've received. It was Mrs. Halifax's request that skilled nursing visits be made each time at 9am. The nurse responded that, although she was unable to adhere to a set appointment for her visits, she would make every effort to schedule Mr. Halifax's visits before noon. By trying to respond to her preferences and priorities, the nurse helped Mrs. Halifax maintain a sense of control and feel good about the home health services they were receiving.

*Show a caring attitude toward the patient and his family.* When asked their impressions of healthcare experiences, many people remember an emotional dimension of their care rather than the technical expertise of the nurse. They mention someone who noticed their personal concerns and "really seemed to care." When Mr. Halifax spoke of his depression over his chronic, disabling health disease, the nurse listened attentively, without giving false reassurances or discounting his feelings. Mr. Halifax felt his feelings of depression and anger had been validated and that the nurse was really concerned about him.

*Deal effectively with patients and caregivers who are angry or upset.* As you know, the burden of illness and accompanying anxiety can strain a patient's or caregiver's coping mechanisms to the breaking point, triggering irritability or anger. One day, the nurse arrived to find Mrs. Halifax angry and upset about a missed home health aide visit. By dealing with Mrs. Halifax in a calm manner, helping to solve her problem and fixing what went wrong, the nurse went a long way toward improving Mrs. Halifax's satisfaction with the agency's services.

## CONCLUSION

In conclusion, patient satisfaction is now recognized as an important outcome measure for quality of care. As a nurse, you are with the patients day in and day out and play a vital role in promoting patient satisfaction. You are in a pivotal position to influence patients' attitudes, perceptions, and memorable impressions of their home health experience.

You are your patient's advocate and your home health agency's best marketing representative. Patients and their families rely mainly on you for assistance, understanding, and support. By demonstrating a caring attitude, recognizing patients as individuals, responding to their fears and anxieties, and doing your best to solve their problems, you can improve patient satisfaction, contribute to reduced costs by reducing patient problems, and promote more positive clinical outcomes.

---

**BIBLIOGRAPHY**

McHann, M.E. *How to Promote Quality Care for Home Health Patients* video. Nursing Videos 1994.
Stricklin, M.L.V. "Home care Consumers Speak Out on Quality," *Home Healthcare Nurse,* Vol 11, Num 6, June 1993.

# Discharge Planning and Quality Assurance

*Marjorie McHann, RN, BS*

Quality assurance... it's one of the biggest issues of the nineties for the home health industry. Why is quality assurance needed especially now in home health care? There are several reasons:

- As a result of DRGs and "quicker but sicker" hospital discharges, the acuity level of home health care patients is rising. With sicker patients and fewer resources, home health agencies are struggling to maintain standards of quality patient care.
- Medicare and other third-party payers are imposing greater reimbursement restrictions on home health agencies. An agency must prove not only that it is providing quality care, but that the care it provides is worth the cost.
- The increasing consumer rights movement in the United States has focused a greater emphasis on quality assurance. Increasing demand for quality services by consumers has forced home health agencies to develop programs to improve quality in care delivery.

All this comes at a time when home health agencies have fewer resources to provide more services to more people who are more seriously ill. Thus, agencies must constantly face cost containment and reimbursement issues and at the same time must attempt to assure the quality of services provided.

The two main concerns of quality assurance are the quality of the services provided and the effectiveness of the services provided. Discharge planning is one of the most important ways to promote cost-effective quality patient care. Discharge planning is a

| Nursing Activities that Promote Effective Discharge Planning |
| --- |
| 1. Accurate assessment of needs and resources<br>2. Early implementation of the discharge plan<br>3. Patient and family involvement<br>4. Using the nursing process<br>5. Coordination of care<br>6. Appropriate patient education<br>7. Effective nursing documentation |

systematic, coordinated process that facilitates continuity of patient care. The purpose of the discharge planning process is to assure that the highest quality of care possible is rendered on a continuous basis.

Reimbursement, accreditation, and professional organizations alike recognize discharge planning as an important component of quality patient care:

- Medicare and other third-party payors recognize discharge planning as an important part of quality care. If adequate discharge planning is not evident in the patient's medical record, reimbursements may be cut.

- Accrediting organizations such as JCAHO and CHAPS also recognize discharge planning as part of high-quality care. Accreditation standards mandate that appropriate discharge planning be done for home health patients and be documented in the medical record. This quality assurance standard is a key factor in the accreditation decision process.

- The American Nurses Association recognizes the importance of discharge planning in the delivery of quality patient care. In its *Standards of Home Health Nursing Practice*, the ANA emphasizes the use of discharge planning to promote continuity of care for home health patients.

As you can see, there is a definite link between discharge planning, quality care, cost containment, and reimbursement. So how does this affect you, the home health nurse? Home health nurses have always been concerned about the quality of care their patients received. But now, more than ever, quality care also means cost-effective care.

As a nurse, you play a vital role in the discharge planning process:

- Judging the assets and limitations of the patient
- Planning for continuity of care upon discharge from the agency, and

- Coordinating needed individual, family, agency, and community resources to implement the discharge plan.

By doing effective discharge planning for your patients, you can help maintain quality patient care, promote better patient outcomes, and insure more cost-effective patient care.

Remember, your home health agency and your patients are depending on you to do appropriate discharge planning to help contain costs and promote quality patient care.

# CHAPTER 6

# Legal Issues

# Legal Implications of Home Health Care

*Helen Creighton, JD, RN*

*Law for the Nurse Manager: Legal Implications of Home Health Care,*
by Helen Creighton, JD, RN. Reprinted with permission
from *Nursing Management* (Vol 18 No 2) February, 1987 issue.

With Medicare's diagnosis-related groups (DRGs) forcing patients out of the hospital sooner and sicker, home health care agencies are trying frantically to cope with heavier patient loads. Needs include more nurses, more time to care for patients, and more money for patient care.

The problem has legal implications for nurses and nursing. While no major cases against home health nurses have been litigated as yet, they will emerge, for malpractice litigation is certain to affect this area of nursing.

*First, hospitals and home health care agencies must look at nurses' education and experience.* Are the nurses associate degree, diploma, baccalaureate graduates? Are they clinical specialists? Have they had education and experience in public health? Have they taken courses in sociology, psychology, cross-cultural relationships, etc.? It does make a difference whether or not the nurses are well prepared to cope with the patient physiologically (such matters as vital signs, edema, difficulty in eating, walking, talking, presence of pain, stage of the illness, etc.) and psychosocially (the economic problems and the spiritual factors involved in the patients' care). The nurses must be proficient in high-tech procedures: patients on respirators, patients of hyperalimentation, patients on intravenous therapy including blood transfusions are among those found in the home health care setting.

Home health care nurses must not accept any assignment for which they are not prepared by education and experience. Prior to undertaking a high-tech assignment, nurses should review the registry's or agency's protocol for handling the equipment and also how to obtain back-up devices. They also should review the registry's or agency's policies and procedures, and their job description.

Home health care nurses should make certain that the registry or agency is licensed by the state, well-administered and experienced. Only such registries and agencies which legally protect the patient can be depended upon to protect the nurse in the event of legal problems. The home health nurse is well advised to carry professional liability insurance which will supplement that carried by the registry or agency.[1]

*Second, the nursing assessment including the physiological, social-psychological, economic and spiritual factors must be on the chart.* "If it is not on the chart, it is not done" is the legal axiom. The patient not only has to receive needed physiological care, but the family or significant others also must be taught how to assist the patient with care *and* how to meet emergencies that may arise.

In addition, as the old adage states: "Every man's home is his castle." In the hospital, the nurse renders care under hospital rules and regulations to which the patient and family must adjust. In home health care, the nurse must adjust to the family home/apartment which may vary significantly in its cleanliness, space, and availability of resources. How thoroughly middle class the majority of nurses are is seldom realized until they enter a home too poor to have table salt available or so elite they greet the nurse as another paid servant. Some people never were good housekeepers at 27 years; they did not improve by 47 or 57 and at 77 and 87 years their housekeeping leaves much to be desired. Some people live in mice, rat, and roach-infested dwellings. Some people are as concerned that you give Puddy, the cat, or Carmel Jo, the dog, his meal as they are that you give them a much-needed injection and dressing change. Other people have a cup of morning coffee sitting over the pilot light on the stove, to refresh "their nurse."

Home health care requires a social-psychological understanding of people, their families and friends. One inner-city 84-year-old couple lived together in an apartment building. The wife was bedridden with multiple complications of age, arthritis, and heart disease. The husband was the manager of the building. Their son brought a pan of food once a day and handed it to the nurse — taking care to touch nothing due to the bedbug-roach problem. Initially, the nurse merely thanked him for his kindness (this was their only food for the day). Several days later she "wondered" if he could bring a little milk for his mother, and then, later, some fruit juice. Gradually, this couple's diet was improved. Eventually, the son came with an added piece of cake for his mother's birthday — and, yes, he was willing to pay for an exterminator twice a month to improve the vermin problem. To be sure, other agencies and their church were contacted for assistance, but family relations were improved and needs were met by kindness and "appreciation"of the son's efforts rather than adverse criticisms.

In another instance, a 90-year-old crippled minister's widow, at the encouragement of a home health nurse, wrote a short series of African children's stories (recalled from bygone years as a missionary) that were published. This gave her new status with her comfortably well-to-do daughter who was much interested in the Pen Women's Group. From being left alone hours at a time and not mentioned to friends, "Mother" gained recognition, visitors and whole new social-psychological surroundings which added joy to her life. Good public relations not only helps the patient and family, but it does prevent and lessen lawsuits, the leading cause of which, according to the Medical Malpractice Commission, is poor public relations.

Many, many home health care patients are in dire economic straits and depend upon the nurse to know and contact community agencies which may assist in meeting their needs. The nurse must work closely with a social worker who, too, may have a case overload. Many patients do not realize that they are eligible to receive food stamps, or that they can get dressings for cancer lesions from the Cancer Society. There also may be local projects such as HOPE (Helping Old People Enthusiastically) in DeSoto County, Arcadia, Florida 33821, which will shop for people, take them to the doctor's or dentist's office, do a bit of needed housework, make minor household repairs, etc.[2]   Such organizations can be of tremendous assistance to the home health care patient.

Then, too, nurses should know the spiritual preference (if any) of their patient in order to contact them. Sometimes, the minister, priest or rabbi chooses to coordinate his call with that of the nurse. Other times the church or synagogue has a service or variety of services (food, clothing, visitors, etc.) which supplement the patient's resources.

*Third, the nursing judgement of the home health care nurse must be an appropriate response to the nursing assessment.* If the tranquilizer prescribed by the physician causes the patient to be very depressed and withdrawn while lessening his/her agitation, the home health nurse must contact the physician, describe the untoward side effects, and get another medicine prescribed which will lessen the agitation without such severe side effects. If the patient requires sterile petroleum jelly gauze dressings for an area where radiation for cancer has caused blood supply failure leaving an open lesion, the nurse must consult with the physician to write a prescription so that such dressings available from central supply through the hospital pharmacy will be paid for by the patient's insurance carrier. (The cost thereof is high and the same are not readily available elsewhere). Since the American Association of Blood Banks has approved home transfusions, by overseeing blood transfusions in the home the home health care nurse can help the patient avoid the problem of and expense of a trip to the hospital.

Home health nurses need an excellent "listening ear." The families of patients are often worn down from constant caregiving and need to unburden themselves to a good listener who can appreciate their tiredness, confinement and stress — even though they do love the patient.[3] To my knowledge, we do not have a program comparable to England's "Six Weeks In and Six Weeks Out" which provides families with certain intermittent relief for caring for the long-term patient. (Under that program, the family takes the patient to a rehabilitation-caring facility for six weeks; the discharge slip is given at the time of the patient's admission. When the family takes the patient home at the end of six weeks, a readmission slip for the patient in six weeks is provided). Such a scheme provides a change for both patient and family.

Nursing judgement, an appropriate response by the nurse to his or her nursing assessment, lessens the chance of a lawsuit whether due to the commission or omission of some act.

*Fourth, documentation is of prime importance for the home health care nurse.* Home health nurses must be especially careful of the words they use. They need to know how the insurer defines "homebound" and "intermittent" or "ambulatory." In some instances, nurses may not use "ambulatory" as the insurer interprets that to mean the patient can manage without a home health nurse.

The Ohio Nurses Association publishes a most helpful document entitled "Documenting Home Care" which the reader may obtain.[4] It contains sample sheets which may be used: Family Information, Initial Assessment/History, Guidelines for Initial Assessment/History, Medical Orders, Controlled Drugs, Medication Sheet, Daily Activity/Treatment, Nursing Care Plan and Nurse Progress Notes. The home health nurse who uses this or comparable documentation has a legally sound record of patient care. When the case is completed, the record should be kept by the nurse or by the registry or home health care agency. For the benefit of the patient and all medical and nursing personnel connected with the patient's care it is important that the nurse keep adequate and accurate records. As the ANA Code states, "The nurse safeguards the client's right to privacy by judiciously protecting information of a confidential nature." The chart also provides proof of service rendered for the third party reimbursement.

After the home care nurse's assessment, Bernzweig advises that a detailed and individualized care plan be signed by the physician — care should not be continued beyond the assessment phase if a care plan has not been approved by a doctor.[5] The home health nurse should know precisely what medications and patient care he or she is expected to give at every visit. In addition such nurse should make certain that he or she has standing orders for handling complications. It is important to note all verbal orders in the chart as well as the substance of any telephone call that relates to changes in the patient's condition and care. The home health care agency should have 24-hour telephone coverage and the nurse must make certain her message to the supervisor or physician is delivered and acted upon.

Documentation must be complete, it must be timely (concurrent with patient care given), and the chart properly identified with the patient's name, diagnosis, date (including the year), physician and nurse. Documentation may mean that a home health nurse finds it necessary to document one reimbursable task, while also performing other duties that are not covered by insurance. Some home health care nurses put in extra time without extra pay just to give patients and families the care they need. Documentation written at the time of the assessment, evaluation or activity is the best evidence of what transpired and is basic to avoiding litigation and winning lawsuits that do occur.

*Fifth, nursing intervention means recording all the various activities you carry out in rendering care to the patient or on his behalf.* On a ventilator-dependent patient, the care which you give to maintain a clear airway, the turning you do to prevent skin breakdown and pneumonia, the passive range-of-motion exercises that you do to relieve pain, the contacting of the physical therapist, occupational therapist, the speech therapist, the dietician, the pulmonary clinical specialist, the clergyman, and others to participate in the health care all have to be recorded. The results of their intervention as it affects the nursing care and its plan have to be noted. What did the nurse do? Why did the nurse engage in this activity? When? What was the patient's and/or family's response? Detailed recording of the nurse's care is necessary to recovering reimbursement for the same and to prevent litigation based on omission of needed care as well as commissions of careless nursing care.

*Sixth, patient and family teaching must be recorded and is central to adequate and good nursing care in the home.* If a home health nurse omits teaching a patient's family how to perform a procedure, it may not get done and if there is resulting harm to the patient, a lawsuit may ensue. One cannot assume the patient teaching was carried out in the hospital. The patient and family are lay people not familiar with sterile technique in suctioning a tracheostomy or flushing a catheter or clearing tubing of air, nor are they familiar with techniques for giving or finding special equipment or food for special diets. Mizuki records an excellent example of the steps needed to help a ventilator-dependent patient go home safely and indicates the follow-through instructions and teaching for which the home health care nurse is responsible.[6]

There a patient with acute intermittent porphyria (AIP), after a complicated nine months in medical intensive care, was transferred to a step-down unit, and then sent home while still ventilator-dependent. The pulmonary clinical specialist provided guidelines for the project. Because of his tracheostomy, the patient communicated by lip and head movements, and he retained bladder and bowel control. He was on a low-calcium, low-potassium, high-carbohydrate diet. Maintaining a clear airway was the first thing taught the wife and her sister. Then prevention of skin breakdown and pneumonia were taught. The procedure for tracheostomy care was taught. The nurse arranged for the delivery of a portable ventilator and a motorized wheelchair as well as a suction machine and bag resuscitator. The physical therapist reviewed the range-of-motion exercise (PROM) with the family and the dietician reviewed the patient's diet with them. Since the patient's insurance would allow 24-hour nursing at home, the appropriate agency was contacted. The social worker, given a list of supplies needed at home, determined which ones the insurance would cover and the nurse had to price other supplies at drug stores and other sources. Prescriptions written by the physician were filled. A daily schedule for meals, bath, PROM exercises, tracheostomy care, sitting in a chair, and naps was planned and posted where the patient and all personnel could use it in his care. The home health nurse had to reinforce the teaching done in the hospital and reteach as necessary in addition to rendering patient care. The home health care nurse contacted the patient's church and a volunteer agency which supplied volunteers to assist the family with various chores and provide company for the patient while the wife and her sister had some much-needed time off. A detailed record of patient teaching is evidence when brought to court that the patient/family were taught how to give the necessary nursing care. There is a need for good communication between the hospital nursing teaching team and the home health care teaching team to be certain that essential material is not omitted.

Articles on Special Teams in Home Care,[7] Safety Precautions in Home Chemotherapy, and Antibiotic Therapy at Home[8] found in the *American Journal of Nursing* familiarize the home health nurse with the special problems in these areas which if mishandled could lead to litigation. As Weinstein states, the objective of home health teaching is to: reduce frequency and number of hospitalizations, reduce the incidence of infection, prevent and recognize serious complications and take appropriate action, maximize performance of activities of daily living, and increase and promote compliance with the medical regimen.[9] Whatever leads to better and more satisfactory nursing care of patients leads to a diminution in the possibility of a lawsuit.

*Seventh, supervision in home health nursing is most important to be certain that nurses are properly prepared and experienced and carrying out their duties despite stressful situations and a heavy case load.*

Documentation must be reviewed to prevent acts of omission or commission that could lead to a lawsuit or lack of reimbursement for the care rendered. Since home health care nurses work alone with minimal supervision, close check must be maintained to ascertain no impaired nurses have slipped into the work force. Impaired nurses often seek positions where minimal supervision allows them to mask their problem. Needless to say, the deteriorating job performance associated with the impaired nurse may be a source of litigation.

In summary, while no major cases against home health nurses have been litigated as yet (August 1986), they will emerge, for malpractice litigation is certain to affect this area of nursing. To prevent such lawsuits, home health nurses need education not only in the physiological aspects of nursing care, but also in social-psychological factors, economic factors and community resources available to help patients and the spiritual factors that may be pertinent. The home health nurse's assessment, appropriate judgement, documentation, intervention, and patient/family teaching must be recorded accurately, timely and in necessary detail as evidence of his/her work in event of litigation. To prevent losses in litigation and reimbursement through negligence, reasonable supervision must also be provided.

---

**REFERENCES**

1. Bernzweig, E., "Avoiding Legal Pitfalls of Home Care," *RN*, 49:49, August, 1986.
2. Southwell, A.R., Adm. Asst. to Director, HOPE Project, DeSoto Co., Arcadia, Florida 33821.
3. Koop, C.E., "Families Caring for Disabled Need Long-term Support," *Hospital Progress*, 67:52-4, July-August, 1986. Discussion of Katie Beckett case where the family took home a 3-year-old on around-the-clock repiratory therapy.
4. Documenting Home Care, Ohio Nurses Association, 4000 E. Main St., Columbus, Ohio, Price $1.50.
5. Note 1, p. 49.
6. Mizuki, J.A., "There is No Place Like Home," *American Journal of Nursing*, 84:647, May 1984.
7. Weinstein, S.M., "Special Teams in Home Health Care," *American Journal of Nursing*, 84:342-5, March, 1984.
8. Schaffner, A., "Safety Precautions in Home Chemotherapy," *American Journal of Nursing*, 84:346-7, March, 1984.
9. Note 7, p. 343.

# Can You Meet the National Standard of Care in Home Health Nursing?

*Nancy I. Connaway, RN, MSN, JD*

Are you a new graduate who is feeling the pressure of caring for complex patients in an acute care unit? Are you unable to give "good" nursing care because your supervisor expects more than you can deliver? Are you an older nurse, returning to the field after raising a family or pursuing other personal goals? If so, you may well be among the hundreds of nurses who are looking at home health care and seeing regular hours, fewer patients, and fewer pressures. Surely, it's the place to be! Before you switch to home health nursing, however, try to view the whole picture. Consider the role, your abilities, and the new national standard of nursing care by which your actions will be measured.

*The independent nature of home health nursing creates potential legal concerns for even the most experienced nurse.* When a patient is cared for at home, nursing supervision and support are at a distance. Since physician contact normally takes place by telephone, every day's nursing action often must be based on a doctor's verbal orders. Nurses who are not sure about current treatment procedures, medication administration protocols, or teaching needs appropriate to various disease processes will quickly find themselves at risk when peers or supervisors are not readily available for consultation.

*Intervention by the patient, the family, and part-time caregivers all affect the caregiving process.* Home health nursing has pressures that are unique in the health care delivery system. Nursing case managers find themselves setting limits for the noncompliant patient and counseling families who intervene to the patient's detriment whenever health care personnel are not present. If the patient's needs exceed the service capability of a single home health agency, the nursing manager must coordinate intermittent care visits as well as the continuous care provided by all health care specialties in order to provide a comprehensive plan of care.

*Hi-tech nursing is the rule rather than the exception.* The institution of diagnosis-related groups (DRGs) and the prospective payment system (PPS) for hospitals has had a profound effect on discharging patients from hospitals to home health care. As a direct effect, older patients who need increased medical-surgical nursing care are being admitted to home care. Previous nursing regimens that called for patient assessment, monitoring, and teaching now include advanced hands-on skills. As an indirect effect of PPS and the national focus on home care as an alternative system of delivering care, younger patients are now being routinely admitted to home health agencies. Infant apnea monitoring, ventilation support, and hyperalimentation therapies for all age groups are now routine home-care procedures.

*Home health nurses must now meet a national standard of care; no longer does the legal standard of care for nursing practice vary according to the locale.* At one time, legal authorities accepted a variation in skill among members of the medical, nursing, and ancillary health professions. Citing unsophisticated communication and transportation systems throughout the nation, courts were hesitant to hold community health practitioners in rural areas to the same standards of care as practitioners in urban areas. With the advancement of communication and transportation systems, however, legal authorities are increasingly rejecting the "locality rule" as a reason to protect nonurban practitioners in negligence suits; within each professional class, regardless of setting, courts now recognize a national standard when assessing the quality of patient care.

Two recent cases illustrate the new rule. In 1979, in the case of *Morrison v McNamara,* 407 A2d 555 (DC 1979) DC Circuit Court of Appeals, a patient who complained of discomfort and dizziness fainted and sustained permanent injury when a lab technician failed to place him an a prone position to obtain a urethral smear. Three local physicians, who were presented as expert witnesses, testified that the local standard of care allowed the smear to be obtained in the standing position. They said that judgement, not the standard of care, dictated whether or not the test should be continued once the patient had complained of faintness. However, the patient's attorney argued that the lab technician should not be evaluated according to local practice. The laboratory was nationally certified and marketed its national accreditation to the public. As such, he argued, the laboratory should be held to a national standard of care. To further support his position, the patient's attorney presented an expert witness who practiced more than 1,000 miles away from the laboratory. This expert testified that the nationally accepted medical standard of care required the test to be administered with the patient in a prone or sitting position to avoid faintness as a result of the vasal-vagal reflex. This witness said that the standard of care, not personal judgement, dictated this safeguard in the test protocol. The court, in deciding to support the plaintiff's position, rejected the locality rule and adopted a national standard of care for judging the technician's performance.

The second case, *Wickliffe v Sunrise Hospital, Inc.*, 706 P2d 1383 (Nev 1985), is one of several that have established national standards for nursing care. This suit was filed by the parents of Angela Wickliffe, a healthy 13-year-old who died in the recovery room after undergoing surgery to correct scoliosis of the spine. The nursing notes in Angela's medical records immediately postop showed a lapse of 1 hour and 10 minutes between the initial and follow-up vital signs; during that period the child experienced cardiac arrest. A nursing expert witness who was called by the plaintiff's attorney in this case cited recovery room standards for nurses that had been developed by the American College of Utilization Review Physicians and by the Joint Commission on Accreditation of Hospitals. Such standards, she testified, form the basis for a common nursing standard throughout the nation for recovery room care. On appeal, the court agreed, emphasizing that there are national standards for nursing and that a common body of knowledge has been developed through nursing education and training.

Each of these cases illustrates the new national standard for community health nurses. As with the facilities described in *Morrison* and *Wickliffe*, home health agencies are state-licensed, certified according to national Medicare standards, and often accredited by the National League for Nursing. Surveys made by these bodies are uniform in both urban and rural settings, reinforcing the expectation that nurses who practice in home health agencies are measured by uniform standards of care. Common elements in nursing education curriculums and state licensure examinations further support this expectation.

If you are a veteran of home health nursing or simply assessing the field for your next career move, consider the complexities of home care described above in light of legal trends in the nursing field. As with nurses in acute care settings, home health nurses are expected to be knowledgeable and competent in rendering nursing care. The standard for such competence is derived for many sources — from agency procedure manuals to ANA standards of practice.

Home health nursing is a specialty! The best legal defense for home health nurses continues to be a sound base of nursing skills coupled with a broad knowledge of agency procedures and industry protocols. Inexperience or lack of orientation to home care protocols and procedures is no defense when a home health nurse, accused of poor patient care, fails to meet national standards expected of peers in the home health field.

* *Editor's Note: See Appendix C for ANA Standards for Home Health Nursing Practice.*

# Documenting Patient Care in the Home - Legal Issues for Home Health Nurses

*Nancy Connaway, RN, MSN, JD*

Every nurse, at one time or another, complains of the paperwork required for the delivery of patient care. Documentation is stressed in a nurse's first course on Fundamentals of Nursing and in every nursing role thereafter.

Documenting patient care is particularly important for home health agencies. Documentation is the critical factor in meeting state licensure and certification requirements, and it is the basis for Medicare and third-party reimbursement for patient care. Because documentation plays such an important role in maintaining the financial status and cash flow of a home health agency, most in-service programs on charting offered to home care nurses emphasize charting techniques for Medicare reimbursement. It is important, however, for home health nurses and supervisors to remember that the clinical record also serves another important purpose: It is an invaluable legal tool and provides the best evidence that a nurse has met professional standards when delivering patient care.

More attention is currently being focused on home health service because patients are now being discharged form hospitals earlier with substantial needs for continued care. Therefore, it is important to reiterate the legal principles of documentation for home health nurses. Although implementing the prospective payment system has not changed the standard of care owed to the patient by a home care nurse, greater demands for care by larger numbers of individuals will increase the legal exposure for home care providers. This article is the first of a two-part series on legal issues in documentation for the home health nurse.

**Why is clinical documentation important?**
Professionally, documentation maintains the continuity of care for the patient and provides a tool to communicate that care to other team members    Legally, the clinical record preserves the action of health care providers in a permanent form. Years later that record might be utilized to refresh the memory of a witness who must offer testimony about the care provided; it might be consulted to discover the facts pertaining to a claim for poor patient care; or it might be examined by an expert witness who must render an opinion on issues essential to litigation claims.

Because the clinical record contains information that is reduced to writing and entered systematically at or near the time the event occurred, it is the best evidence that the home care nurse met the professional duty owed to the patient.

**What are the legal guidelines for professional charting in any setting?**
Briefly, they are as follows:
- Write legibly and neatly using correct spelling and grammar. The public, and consequently a jury, tends to equate sloppy charting with sloppy care.
- Chart in ballpoint pen only. Pencil lead may be erased, and felt-tip ink may be smudged by water stains.
- Do not leave blank lines or spaces in the nursing notes. Others may wonder what you forgot to write and, therefore, what you forgot to do.
- Authenticate flow-sheet entries by signature and date.
- Never obliterate an entry entirely or use correction fluid to rectify an error. Cross through a mistake, leaving it legible; then enter the correct information below.
- Late entries are legally acceptable additions if labeled as an addendum, signed, and included in the chart.
- Never allow someone else to chart for you or sign your name after nursing entries. Never recopy another's entries.
- Use common abbreviations only; to reference abbreviations use your agency policy and procedure manual.
- Document the nursing process, being sure to include the patient's response to treatment rendered.
- Document communication between team members and physicians, especially if the patient's condition is changing. Document all nursing follow-up to such communication.

## SPECIAL DOCUMENTATION ISSUES FOR HOME HEALTH NURSES

The very nature of home health care presents special documentation issues for the home health nurse.

**Supervision of care is at a distance.** Because patient care is rendered in a number of homes by a multitude of agency personnel, nursing supervision is not continually available on site as the tasks are performed. Supervision may be accomplished by telephone and periodic home visits. Contact and supervision are often responses to a patient complaint.

Regardless of patient care setting, a nursing supervisor is expected, by law, to fulfill the responsibilities of the job description. Primarily, these responsibilities are to delegate nursing care appropriately (ie, a specific nursing task should be given to the appropriate person according to that person's education and experience in performing the task) and to supervise performance of the delegated task to assure safe, effective patient care. Home health nursing supervisors should prepare a document to indicate that all legal obligations have been fulfilled.

Supervisory notes should reflect that:

- Task assignments have been appropriate to the skills of the professionals and nonprofessionals assigned to patient care.
- Care rendered has been delegated or performed within the parameters of the Nurse Practice Act.
- Tasks have been performed in accordance with agency policies and procedures and local standards of care.
- Patient outcome has been responsive to treatment or appropriate actions have been implemented.
- Inappropriate nursing actions have been identified immediately.

**Two or more agencies share patient care.** Sometimes the needs of a patient exceed the service capability of a single home health agency. When this occurs, two or more agencies may share patient care, providing a variety of intermittent visits and/or continuous care to the same patient. Patient care and documentation of a that care in the clinical record must not be compromised because two agencies share patient service.

Documentation issues that must be resolved should address which agency will obtain doctors' orders and maintain the complete clinical record of patient care. This task most often falls to the agency that undertakes billing responsibility for patient care, with the second agency subcontracting to the other for service. Nursing entries should be entered sequentially and should be available to both provider agencies to establish that standards of care have been met.

If continuous care is provided, with one nurse following another into the home, written doctors' orders, care plans, and progress notes should be available in the home. Professional nurses have an affirmative obligation to check doctors' orders prior to rendering skilled care, and the unavailability of the chart and/or doctors' orders is no defense to a claim of negligence if an error causes harm to the patient.

**Obtaining doctors' orders routinely by telephone.**

As home care becomes technically more complex and direct patient treatment increases, the documentation of accurate, individualized doctors' orders is most important.

Although it is accepted practice for RNs to accept doctors' orders by telephone, nurse supervisors should consult the Nurse Practice Act of their jurisdiction to determine if LVNs (LPNs) may also accept doctors' orders by telephone before delegating such a task to them. In all cases, telephone orders should be confirmed in writing by the physician in a timely manner according to the home health licensure law. While telephone orders should be communicated in writing to other non-nurse primary caregivers, one's local Nurse Practice Act should be consulted to determine whether it is acceptable to transmit doctors' orders verbally from one nurse to another without written documentation.

Agency procedures for documenting physicians' orders should include:
- Who may call the physician from the home for orders?
- How will verbal telephone orders be confirmed by the physician?
- How will verbal orders obtained at home be documented for communication to other team members for coordinated care?

Telephone calls to the physician to report patient problems should be a routine documentation responsibility for all nurses. It is especially important to document nursing actions which provide evidence of a follow-up to each call to the physician if the patient's condition is unstable.

**Documenting environmental factors and intervention by family members.**

At least one writer has commented that home health nurses hesitate to document family interventions or to describe environmental factors that affect patient outcome for fear that the family may eventually read the nursing entry (Schipske, 1984). Under other circumstances, nurses may fail to fully describe treatment protocols for fear that the patients' reimbursement will be denied. For instance, documenting a case plan of progressive ambulation may mean Medicare reimbursement denial for the cardiac rehabilitation patient at home.

Legally, sound practice dictates that the nurse document all factors that influence any phase of the nursing process or the outcome of patient care. Providing care below this standard or failing to provide care may be interpreted by others as an act of negligence. Omitting important environmental data or portions of the care plan may indicate that the nurse was negligent in assessing the patient, planning for care, delivering care, or evaluating care.

Therefore, although it is possible that the patient or family may read the chart at some future time, the documentation of environmental data may prove the only defense before a tribunal if a home care nurse is accused of negligent nursing care. Entries about the family or environment should, however, be objective, factual, and directly impact some portion of the nursing process.

**Increased use of part-time personnel.**

As home health agencies become busier, the use of part-time personnel may increase. Persons who work part-time for one or more employers may be unfamiliar with the policies and procedures specific to your agency and thus they may deviate from these guidelines when delivering patient care. Case managers and nursing supervisors should review the documentation of part-time professionals and nonprofessionals alike to make sure that patient care is not being compromised, thereby increasing the legal liability for the caregiver, supervisor, and home care agency. Agency policies and procedures are legally established standards for measuring the adequacy of job performance and patient care (Darling v Charleston Community Memorial Hospital, 1965).

To limit liability, home care supervisors should be certain that:
- Part-time personnel are oriented to the policies and procedures for nursing care, and that such orientation is documented.

- Documentation by part-time caregivers is routinely reviewed to identify any deviations from policy.
- Appropriate follow-up instructions are given and documented to align action with policy.

Documentation of instructions on agency policy and procedures should be included in the individual personnel record rather than in the clinical record unless patient care is at issue.

## Conclusion

Documentation of home health care continues to be the single most important factor in the survival of an agency. It is the ;mechanism through which licensure standing and reimbursement are obtained. However, home health nurses, like all other medical professionals, must also document to provide a legal record verifying that safe, effective care was provided to the patient. Quality assurance measures that address the foregoing issues will assist home health nurses, case managers and supervisors in establishing a written record confirming that the professional standard of care owed to the home care patient has been met. Next month, this column will discuss special documentation concerns for home health nurses: death bed statements, access to the clinical record, and witnessing documents in the patient's home.

---

**BIBLIOGRAPHY**

Schipske G (1984, May). Documenting care for the patient at home. *Coordinator.*
Darling v Charleston Community Memorial Hospital, 33 Ill 2d 325, 211 NE 2d 253 (1965); Burks v Christ Hospital, 19 Ohio St 2d 128, 249 NE 2d 829 (1969).

# Avoiding Professional Negligence: A Review

*Nancy J. Brent, RN, MS, JD*

Although there are many areas of liability that the nurse, including the home healthcare nurse, must be concerned about when practicing nursing, perhaps the most frequent area that comes to the minds of most nurses is that of professional negligence or professional malpractice. This probably occurs because professional negligence is a topic that receives a great deal of coverage in textbooks on law and nursing practice, journal articles, and seminars covering professional practice issues. And, it is an area that is receiving increasing attention from professional liability insurance carriers and professional organizations as well. Recently, the American Nurses' Association has coordinated the establishment of a "National Nurses Claims Data Bank" to provide for compilation of statistics concerning nurses who are named as defendants in lawsuits, the types of suits that are filed against nurses, and other types of information necessary to monitor the increasing numbers of nurses involved in suits concerning their practice.[1] Furthermore, a 1988 study conducted for the American Nurses' Association by a New York-based management consultant and actuary firm to realistically determine claims and losses against nurses in liability suits confirmed that, insofar as *one* insurance underwriter's figures indicated, approximately 1,900 nurses were named in suits during the year, with the average payment to the plaintiff being $145,397.00.[2]

Despite the fact that nurses are being sued in increasing numbers, the American Nurses' Association estimates that only 6.2 RNs in 10,000 will be sued each year, in comparison with 1,800 physicians in 10,000 who will be named as defendants.[3] Even so, it is important for the home healthcare nurse to avoid inclusion in that 6.2 number as much as possible. One way to avoid being named in a professional negligence lawsuit is to understand how the law applies this cause of action to the healthcare provider.

## DEFINITION AND ELEMENTS OF NEGLIGENCE

Negligence is an example of a tort, which is a civil "wrong or injury," other than one that involves a breach of contract where the individual seeks redress in the form of monetary compensation for his injuries or the damages sustained.[4] Negligence can involve acts of omission or commission and is "conduct that falls below the standard established by law for the protection of others against unreasonable risk of harm."[4] In addition to protecting another against an unreasonable risk of harm, the law requires another also to protect the other person from a foreseeable risk of harm. It also holds each individual responsible for his or her own behavior, including negligent behavior.

For conduct to be negligent, however, the law requires that four major elements be satisfied (i.e., proven in court) before a plaintiff can be successful. Those elements include:

1. A duty or obligation to adhere to a certain standard or conduct himself or herself in a certain manner must exist;
2. A failure or "breach" of that standard must occur;
3. The failure or "breach" must have caused the injury or the damages suffered (often called the "proximate cause" or "legal cause" of the damages); and
4. Damages or injuries are sustained that are recognized and compensable by law.[5]

Last but not least, the law measures a person's overall conduct in an alleged negligent situation by comparing that conduct with what an "ordinary, reasonable, and prudent" person would do in those same or similar circumstances.[5]

## PROFESSIONAL NEGLIGENCE

The definition and elements of negligence presented thus far concern nonprofessional persons. When a person possesses additional skills, knowledge, or expertise in a certain area, such as nurses, physicians, and lawyers, the law applies the basic principles of negligence to them but adjusts the overall standard of conduct expected in the particular situation to that of another professional in the same group. Thus, when a home healthcare nurse is allegedly negligent, causing injury to a patient, the same elements must be proven by that injured patient, but the nurse's conduct would be compared with that of an "ordinary, reasonable and prudent" home healthcare nurse in the same or similar circumstances in the same or similar community. The same or similar community standard is, in reality, a "national standard,"[5] meaning that the home healthcare nurse must be familiar with, and conduct patient care in accordance with, standards promulgated by national professional associations such as The National League for Nursing, The American Nurses' Association, or The American Association of Neuroscience Nurses.

In addition to adhering to national standards of care when providing care hopefully to avoid the rendering of negligent care, knowledge of these standards are important because of a unique aspect of any trial involving professional negligence. Because the jury is composed of lay persons (i.e., individuals unfamiliar with medical and nursing practice) an expert witness must be used to establish the standard of care and give an opinion to the jury as to whether the nurse on trial deviated from that standard of care. Because an expert witness can in many instances come from any part of the country and must speak to "what is customary and usual in the profession,"[5] these standards are used by the expert in formulating his or her opinion.

## THE HOME HEALTHCARE NURSE AND PROFESSIONAL NEGLIGENCE SUITS

Relatively few, if any, suits to date have been filed against home healthcare nurses and their employers.[6] How long this will continue to be true, however, is not known. Rather than simply bask in the freedom from inclusion in lawsuits, home healthcare nurses and their employers can vigorously work to continue this unusual position.

One way in which the home healthcare nurse and his or her employer can continue this status is through the development of a good risk management and quality assurance program, especially in the area of potential patient care liabilities, such as delegation of tasks, consent and refusal of treatment, and safety of the patient and the family in the home when care is provided.[7]   Home healthcare nurse administrators need to develop and implement clear and concise job descriptions, policies, and procedures for nursing staff. Support for home healthcare nurses to attend continuing education programs concerning updates in delivering care in the home, and concerning potential legal liabilities, is also important. And, as is true in the acute care setting, adequate numbers of competent staff, including supervisors, is essential.

Another approach to liability avoidance is the establishment and maintenance of good, open lines of communication between the patient and family and the home healthcare nurse and agency. Although it is true that if one experiences a serious injury as a result of a nurse's negligence, little or nothing may prevent that individual from seeking redress in the court, it is also true that the decision to litigate is based on many factors other than an injury alone. One such factor may be how the patient and the family perceived the home healthcare nurse and his or her employer as treating them during the course of providing care. If seen as caring and compassionate healthcare providers, although the decision may still be made to sue, it is made with a different emotional stance than if the decision is based on a wealth of anger and unhappiness generally with the care provided and the manner in which the person was treated.

Experienced anger and unhappiness can also be carried into the litigation process itself, resulting in a "do or die" stance where no settlement or compromise can take place. That approach is not helpful to an already expensive, adversarial process, which one state supreme court justice has described as having no true winners, regardless of the outcome.[8]

Could it be that easy, then, to avoid unnecessary involvement in a lose-lose situation like litigation by simply delivering care consistent with "what is customary and usual in the profession" and do so in a humane, caring, and compassionate way? Perhaps that is what home healthcare nurses have been doing and is one reason why few suits have been filed against them. If it is one of the reasons, it should be continued. If the home healthcare nurse and the agency hadn't thought about this approach as a good risk management principle, it sounds like it is worth a try.

---

## REFERENCES

1. DataBase monitors liability claims. *Continuing Care* (January 1989), 24-25: American Nurses' Association. *Nurses & Hospitals, Partners in Prevention.* A Public Service Announcement Poster, 1990.

2. Study of liability claims releases first findings. *Am Nurse* 1988: 20(2):33.
3. How likely is a lawsuit? *Am J Nurs* 1990: 90(1): 42.
4. Black HC: *Black's Law Dictionary*. 5th ed. St. Paul, MN: West Publishing Company, 1983: 774.
5. Keeton WP, ed: *Prosser and Keeton on the Law of Trots*. 5th ed. St. Paul, MN: West Publishing Company, 1984: 164.
6. Crompton DE: Alternative delivery systems; risk management and the law. *Columbia University Law Rev* 1987; 17: 357-71.
7. Brent NJ: Risk management in home care: focus on patient care liabilities. *Loyola University of Chicago Law J* 1989; 20:775-95.
8. Neely R: *How Courts Govern America*. New Haven: Yale University Press, 1981: xiv.

# Delegation and Supervision of Patient Care

*Nancy J. Brent, RN, MS, JD*

Home healthcare nursing practice is unique in many ways. One of its distinctive characteristics is the delivery of nursing care in the home. Home healthcare nurses must be innovative and independent in the provision of care to patients in such a setting. They must also be astute delegators and supervisors of patient care to others on the home healthcare team.

Because the home healthcare team is composed of nursing professionals (defined for this column as registered nurses [RNs] and licensed practical nurses [LPNs]) and paraprofessionals (those who are *not* licensed but provide aspects of nursing care, such as home health aides or homemakers), the home healthcare nurse must ensure that any delegation and supervision is consistent within the law(s) that impact on delegation and supervision.

## DELEGATION

Delegation has been defined as the transfer of authority by one person to another and entrusting the one delegated with the power to act for that person.[1] Thus, when the nurse delegates patient care to another, there is a decision that the person asked to "stand in his or her stead" is trustworthy to do so. Trust in the other individual is not enough, however, for the nurse who delegates must conform to certain *legal* parameters.

One legal parameter of delegation is being certain that the delegating is done in a nonnegligent manner. When assigning another to perform certain patient care, the home healthcare nurse must be certain that he or she selects the person with a clear understanding of his or her own skills and abilities. This is important so that no foreseeable, unreasonable risk of harm comes to the patient because of the other person's incompetency, lack of skills, or inability to perform that which is delegated. Should an injury occur as a result of the care given, the home healthcare nurse-delegator's decision will be compared to what other ordinary, reasonable, and prudent home healthcare nurses would have done in similar circumstances.

A second concern for the home healthcare nurse-delegator is ensuring that any delegation is consistent with the state nursing act. Delegation is often defined in state nurse practice acts or its rules or regulations. For example, in the Rules for Administration of the Illinois Nursing Act of 1987, Illinois defines delegation as "...assignment of tasks...or professional responsibilities...to another in which the supervisor holds the other individual responsible and accountable for performance while maintaining accountability for the assigned tasks and professional responsibilities."[2]

Likewise, Minnesota and Wisconsin contain language in their respective practice acts and/or rules and regulations that affect delegation.[3] In fact, the American Nurse's Association has recommended that a definition of "professional nursing practice" and "technical nursing practice" include language concerning the delegation and supervision of patient care.[4]

In addition to defining delegation, practice statutes may also define *what* can be delegated, the circumstances under which delegation can occur, and to whom delegated care can be given. Illinois' rules state that an RN can delegate a "task" only to those who are qualified by education and experience. In contrast, a "professional responsibility" can only be delegated to those who are licensed to perform them.[5]


## SUPERVISION

Supervision is defined as the act of "overseeing" an individual or process.[6] It requires the supervisor to continue to manage and monitor those individuals or the work at hand.

Supervision in home healthcare is no exception. The home healthcare nurse who supervises others on the home healthcare team must do so with an ever-vigilant eye toward the ultimate goal — providing quality nursing care to the patient in the home setting.

Potential liabilities for the home healthcare nurse who supervises is not unlike those already discussed in relation to delegation. Supervision must be done in a nonnegligent manner. That includes, but is not limited to, being available to those who are supervised; performing supervisory responsibilities in a manner consistent with particular standards of care; and performing supervisory responsibilities in conformity with what other ordinary, reasonable, and prudent home healthcare nurses would do when performing that role.

As with delegation, many nurse practice acts also define the particulars of supervision in the delivery of nursing care. Illinois defines "supervision" as monitoring and guiding (another), with accountability for what is delegated and supervised remaining with the supervisor.[7] Wisconsin requires the nurse who supervises delegated nursing acts to observe and monitor the activities of those supervised and provide direction and assistance to those individuals.[8]

## IMPLICATIONS FOR HOME HEALTHCARE NURSES

Before delegating or supervising any patient care, the home healthcare nurse should:

- review agency policies concerning delegation and supervision;
- be familiar with the state nurse practice act and its rules and regulations concerning delegation and supervision;
- use other RNs and LPNs consistent with their respective abilities *and* within the legal parameters of their practice as defined in the state practice act;
- use others on the home healthcare team for those aspects of care not requiring an RN or LPN to perform;
- know the skills, strengths, weaknesses, and abilities of those supervised and delegated; and
- perform the supervisory role in a careful, nonnegligent manner.

Patient care assignments cannot be taken lightly. A risk management approach — preventing problems before they arise — is the best defense.[9] Liability for improper delegation or supervision, whether because of allegations of professional negligence or a violation of the state nurse practice act, is a concern for all home healthcare nurses who make daily decisions concerning patient care.

## REFERENCES

1. Henry Campbell Black. *Black's Law Dictionary.* 6th Ed. St. Paul, MN: West Publishing, 1991, p. 294.
2. 14 Ill. Reg. 10035, 1300.10 (e) (1990).
3. Minnesota Statutes Annotated, Section 148.171 *et seq* (1955), *as amended*; Wisconsin Administrative Code, Chapter N6 *et seq* (1983) *as amended.*
4. American Nurses' Association. *Suggested State Legislation: Nursing Practice Act, Nursing Disciplinary Diversion Act, Prescriptive Authority Act.* Kansas City, MO: American Nurses Association, 1990, pp. 8 - 10.
5. 14 Ill. Reg. 10035, 1300-42 (1990).
6. *The Random House College Dictionary.* Revised Ed. New York: Random House, 1984, p. 1320.
7. 14 Ill. Reg. 10035, 1300-10 (c) (1990).
8. Wisconsin Administrative Code, Chapter N6, N 6.03 (3) (a)-(d) (1983), *as amended* (Standards of Practice for Registered Nurses).
9. Brent NJ. Risk Management in Home Health Care: Focus on Patient Care Liabilities. *Loyola University of Chicago Law Journal* 1989; 20(3): 775-795.

# Appendices

# Homecare Patient Bill of Rights

Home care clients have a right to be notified in writing of their rights and obligations before treatment begins. The client's family or guardian may exercise the client's rights when the client has been judged incompetent. Home care providers have an obligation to protect and promote the rights of their clients, including the following rights.

## CLIENTS AND PROVIDERS HAVE A RIGHT TO DIGNITY AND RESPECT

Home care clients and their formal caregivers have a right to not be discriminated against based on race, color, religion, national origin, age, sex, or handicap. Furthermore, clients and caregivers have a right to mutual respect and dignity, including respect for property. Caregivers are prohibited from accepting personal gifts and borrowing from clients.

**Clients have the right:**
- to have relationships with home care providers that are based on honesty and ethical standards of conduct;
- to be informed of the procedure they can follow to lodge complaints with the home care provider about the care that is, or fails to be, furnished, and regarding a lack of respect for property. (To lodge complaints with us call _____);
- to know about the disposition of such complaints;

reprisal for having done so; and
- to be advised of the telephone number and hours of operation of the state's home health "hot line," which receives complaints or questions about local home care agencies. The hours are _____ and the number is _____.

## DECISIONMAKING

**Clients have the right:**
- to be notified about the care that is to be furnished, the types (disciplines) of the caregivers who will furnish the care, and the frequency of the visits that are proposed to be furnished;
- to be advised of any change in the plan of care before the change is made;
- to participate in the planning of the care and in planning changes in the care, and to be advised that they have the right to do so;
- to be informed in writing of rights under state law to make decisions concerning medical care including the right to accept or refuse treatment and the right to formulate advance directives;
- to be informed in writing of policies and procedures for implementing advance directives including any limitations if the provider cannot implement an advance directive on the basis of conscience;
- to have health care providers comply with advance directives in accordance with state law requirements;
- to receive care without condition on, or discrimination based on, the execution of advance directives; and
- to refuse services without fear of reprisal or discrimination.

The home care provider or the client's physician may be forced to refer the client to another source of care if the client's refusal to comply with the plan of care threatens to compromise the provider's commitment to quality care.

## PRIVACY

**Clients have the right:**
- to confidentiality of information about their health, social, and financial circumstances and about what takes place in the home;

and
- to expect the home care provider to release information only as required by law or authorized by the client.


## FINANCIAL INFORMATION

**Clients have the right:**
- to be informed of the extent to which payment may be expected from Medicare, Medicaid, or any other payor known to the home care provider;
- to be informed of the charges that will not be covered by Medicare;
- to be informed of the charges for with the client may be liable;
- to receive this information, orally and in writing, before care is initiated and within 30 working days of the date the home provider becomes aware of any changes in charges; and
- to have access, upon request, to all bills for service the client has received regardless of whether the bills are paid out-of-pocket or by another party.


## QUALITY OF CARE

**Clients have the right:**
- to receive care of the highest quality;
- in general, to be admitted by a home care provider only if it has the resources needed to provide the care safely and at the required level of intensity, as determined by a professional assessment; a provider with less than optimal resources may nevertheless admit the client if a more appropriate provider is not available, but only after fully informing the client of the provider's limitations and the lack of suitable alternative arrangements; and
- to be told what to do in the case of an emergency.

**The home care provider shall assure that:**
- all medically related home care is provided in accordance with physicians' orders and that a plan of care specifies the services and their frequency and duration; and
- all medically related personal care is provided by an appropriately trained home care aide who is supervised by a nurse or other qualified home care professional.

## CLIENT RESPONSIBILITY

**Clients have the responsibility:**
- to notify the provider of changes in their condition (e.g., hospitalization, changes in the plan of care, symptoms to be reported);
- to follow the plan of care;
- to notify the provider if the visit schedule needs to be changed;
- to inform providers of the existence of, and any changes made to, advance directives;
- to advise the provider of any problems or dissatisfaction with the services provided;
- to provide a safe environment for care to be provided; and
- to carry out mutually agreed responsibilities.


*To satisfy the Medicare certification requirements, the Health Care Financing Administration requires that agencies:
   1.    Give a copy of the Bill of Rights to each patient in the course of the admission process.
   2.    Explain the Bill of Rights to the patient and document that this has been done.
To minimize confusion, NAHC recommends that agencies have clients sign *one form* that shows that the client acknowledges all of the agency's policies and procedures (e.g., release of medical information, billing procedures).

# Generic Quality Screens - Home Health Agency

Reprinted from *Medicare Peer Review Organization Manual,*
Department of Health and Human Services,
Health Care Financing Administration,
Health Standards and Quality Bureau,
Published February 1993.

1. **Adequacy of Intake Evaluation**
   a. Adequate assessment of HHA's capacity to provide the services required for recovery or maximum restoration of function. Assessment to include:
      - History.
      - Physical assessment/functional limits/impairment.
      - Activities of daily living (ADL).
      - Psycho-social (cognitive and affective).
      - Caregiver.
      - Review of medications.
      - Nutritional needs.
      - Environmental risks.
   b. Adequate assessment of physical environment, and capability of caregiver to provide care in the home.
   c. Adequate assessment of patient before or at time of admission, and source of referral to HHA.

2. **Appropriate and Timely Interventions**
   a. Presence of temperature elevation of 100°F oral (101°F rectal), or presence of hypothermia without physician notification within 4 hours from the time detected.
   b. Presence of B.P. reading of < 85 or > 180 systolic, or <

   c. Presence of pulse < 50 (or 45 if the patient is on a beta blocker) or > 120 without physician notification within 4 hours from the time detected.
   d. Presence of other significant changes in signs and symptoms without physician notification within 4 hours from time detected. Examples:
   • Mental status (re: changes in cognitive function or behavior)
   • Loss of function
   • Signs and symptoms of Congestive Heart Failure (CHF), etc.
   e. Appropriate diagnostic services provided on physician's orders.
   f. Abnormal results of diagnostic services addressed and resolved, or the record explains why they are unresolved.
   g. Appropriate intervention if significant change in social support system, including environment.
   h. Appropriate reporting of abuse/neglect.
   i. Timely reporting to physician of lack of family and/or patient compliance

3. **Adequacy of Restorative Care**
   a. Specialty therapies.
      1. Restorative need identified and addressed through assessment, plan, implementation and evaluation.
      2. Presence of therapy plan of care and documentation of therapist's compliance with plan.
      3. Presence of patient education.
   b. Nursing instructions.
      1. Presence of patient education plan and documentation of nursing compliance with the plan.
      2. Documentation in the nursing care plan of coordination of services (interdisciplinary follow-up and reinforcement).
      3. Continual reassessment of patient's needs with referrals to other disciplines as necessary.

4. **Deaths**
   Deaths within 48 hours of transfer to hospital as ascertained from the hospital record

5. **Possible Indications of Secondary Infections**
   a. Temperature elevation > 2 degrees after 72 hours of start

of care.
b.  Any indication of an infection following an invasive procedure

6.  **Issues Related to Patient Care After the Home Health Start of Care**
    a.  Presence of incident with resultant injury or untoward effect.
    b.  Presence of decubitus ulcer.
    c.  Presence of life-threatening complications.
    d.  Adverse drug reaction or medication error.
    e.  Evidence of inappropriate planning and administration of patient care.
    f.  Responsibility for termination of care only when services are no longer required.

7.  **Discharge Plan and Follow-up.**
    Documented plan for appropriate follow-up care and discharge summary to physician(s) of record.

8.  **Adequacy of Care.**
    In the judgement of the professional reviewer, are there any other events/patterns of care that resulted in adverse outcomes that should be evaluated?

    No_____     Yes _____     Explain

# The ANA Home Care Nursing Standards

Reprinted with permission
from *Standards of Home Health Nursing Practice,*
© 1986, American Nurses' Association, Washington, DC.

**Standard I.    Organization of Home Health Services**
All home health services are planned, organized, and directed by a master's-prepared professional nurse with experience in community health and administration.

**Standard II.    Theory**
The nurse applies theoretical concepts as a basis for decisions in practice.

**Standard III.    Data Collection**
The nurse continuously collects and records data that are comprehensive, accurate, and systematic.

**Standard IV.    Diagnosis**
The nurse uses health assessment data to determine nursing diagnoses.

**Standard V.    Planning**
The nurse develops care plans that establish goals. The care plan is based on nursing diagnoses and incorporates therapeutic, preventive, and rehabilitative nursing actions.

**Standard VI.    Intervention**
The nurse, guided by the care plan, intervenes to provide comfort, to restore, improve, and promote health, to prevent complications and sequelae of illness, and to effect rehabilitation.

to interventions in order to determine progress toward goal attainment and to revise the data base, nursing diagnosis, and plan of care.

**Standard VIII. Continuity of Care**
The nurse is responsible for the client's appropriate and uninterrupted care along the health care continuum, and therefore, uses discharge planning, case management, and coordination of community resources.

**Standard IX. Interdisciplinary Collaboration**
The nurse initiates and maintains a liaison relationship with all appropriate health care providers to assure that all efforts effectively complement one another.

**Standard X. Professional Development**
The nurse assumes responsibility for professional development and contributes to the professional growth of others.

**Standard XI. Research**
The nurse participates in research activities that contribute to the profession's continuing development of knowledge of home health care.

**Standard XII. Ethics**
The nurse uses the code for nurses established by the American Nurses' Association as a guide for ethical decision making in practice.